THE COMPLETE BOOK OF
fashion modeling

THE COMPLETE BOOK OF

fashion

BERNIE LENZ Director, Lenz Finishin

From basic fashion and photography modeling techniques for beginners, to expert modeling for stage, runway, tearoom, salon, wholesale, retail, and television—with complete instructions on how to produce your own fashion show, and a full section on model beauty

modeling

chool and Model Agency, Las Vegas, Nevada

with the editorial assistance of Ria Niccoli

Crown Publishers, Inc., New York

To Richard,
who, without taking a lesson,
is a model . . . husband

© 1969, by Bernie Lenz
Library of Congress Catalog Card Number: 68-59486
ISBN: 0-517-501937
Printed in the United States of America
Published simultaneously in Canada by General Publishing Company Limited

Designed by Leonard Cascioli

Fourth Printing, September, 1972

Contents

PREFACE

Every young girl or woman who has a desire to learn modeling should have that opportunity.

She may model for organizations or social events, or she may go into the field professionally, either part-time or full-time. Let her model well and with knowledge.

There should be no difference between the techniques of a big-city model and a small-town model. The only differences would lie in the wishes of those for whom she is modeling. She should understand how a designer would want the clothes shown to an audience. Learn to fit the mood to the fashion show, and know it isn't done to the best advantage without training.

It has been my pleasure to guide, teach, and direct models of all ages. Without exception, the personality of a girl blossoms when she has learned to model and has an opportunity to use this knowledge occasionally. The grace, assurance, and poise the training gives will be an asset throughout your entire life. It is little short of a miracle, the change that comes about through training in the art of modeling.

It is my pleasure to bring you this training in an easy picture-form method. Practice each phase carefully and with a feeling of smoothness.

If you have a desire to continue professionally, may I suggest that you have your self-taught modeling training checked by an expert? There are many experts throughout the country. They can let you know where you need more practice, and what *you* may not see, *they* will.

As an officer of the Modeling Association of America, I have taught my methods of training to many schools throughout the United States. The results have been exceptional, and many of my models have gone on to achieve success in the modeling profession.

The object of this book is to encourage children, teen-agers, and women of all ages to learn to model for their own improvement and enjoyment, even if they never plan to make modeling a career.

This book is an excellent guide for any girl or woman who has ever aspired to become a model. The techniques learned will encourage her to contact her local model agency for an interview. The information in this book will also serve as an invaluable guide for the professional model who wishes to brush up on the latest techniques. The previously trained model is in a position to evaluate her knowledge of modeling and to realize the necessity of always learning new techniques. The professional continues to learn and practice forever.

There are many girls and women who would like to know how to model, yet would never pay for a course until they learn how much this training could do for them. Many of these women will take an interest in professional modeling once they have been inspired and realize that a beautiful model who is well trained makes everything appear easy.

There are techniques to be learned in modeling so that one can become an accomplished model who is very much in demand. If you never model professionally, at least you will learn how to acquire the grace and poise you admire in others.

We know you will be pleased with the results. Good luck!

B. L.

ACKNOWLEDGMENTS

Before I begin, I would like to express my gratitude to all who have helped me in the preparation of this book. Some have helped directly, and many, indirectly. The influence of friends and of people I admire in the modeling profession has increased my knowledge. Without them, the book would not be possible.

The Modeling Association of America and its members from fifty states.

Joy Edelstein, Shore Model Agency, Asbury Park, New Jersey.

Loretta Secret, designer and consultant.

Lenz models, and especially Yvonne Mongeon, Fashion Model Instructor.

Janet Grube and Jo Ann Bolen, Lenz models who posed for illustrations.

Gail Stewart, *Vogue* Fashion Model.

New York model agencies:

Phyllis Chaizel, Bonnie Kid Model Agency

Eileen and Jerry Ford, Ford Model Agency

Frances Gill, Frances Gill Agency

Cye Perkins, Perkins Model Agency

Wilhelmina and Bruce Cooper, Wilhelmina Model Agency

Nina Blanchard, Nina Blanchard Model Agency, Los Angeles.

Nerice Fugate Moore, House of Charm Model Agency, San Francisco.

Stewart Models, Inc., New York

Serendipity Models, New York

Dorothy Lohman Model Agency, New York

To the many European and Oriental models who have worked with me.

Terry Grimes Russell, publicity manager of Clairol, Inc.

Dick and Carlo La Torre, Make-Up Center, Ltd., New York.

Tom Jungman, photographer, New York.

Al Belson, photographer, Las Vegas, Nevada.

Philip Pegler, photographer, New York.

Enny of Italy, Inc., wigs and hairpieces, New York.

A special thank you to all the models represented in the book.

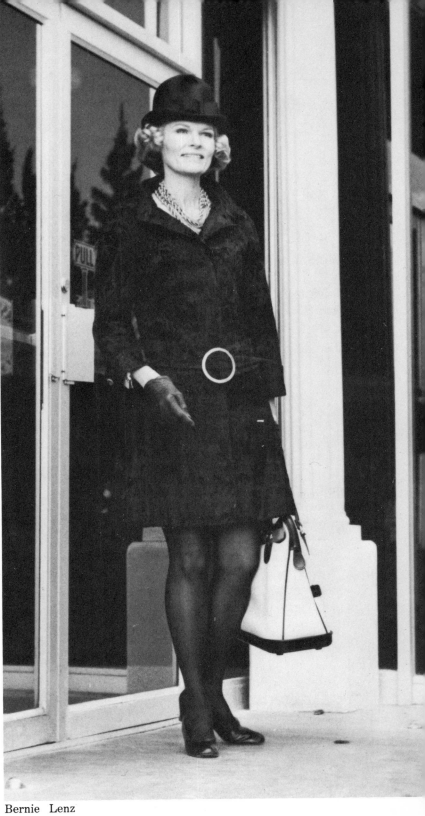

Bernie Lenz

1

THE ADVANTAGES OF BEING A MODEL

You don't have to be particularly beautiful to be a model, and you don't have to belong to any certain age group. Children, teen-agers, single girls, housewives, and grandmothers — there's a place for each of them somewhere within the field. The trick is to find your proper place, and then prepare for it. That's what this book is all about.

The world of modeling is widespread, its citizens are legion, and its advantages are enormous. There's glamour, excitement, money, and opportunity. There's a chance to travel, for those who want to. For those who don't, there's an opportunity to earn money without stepping outside your own town. Best of all, modeling is for everyone.

You can set your sights on stardom or carve a comfortable niche for yourself right in your own community. How far — and how fast — you go is entirely up to you.

In a modeling career, there is literally no limit to the things you can do and the places you can go to. Modeling can open new doors for you everywhere. You'll find opportunities you've never dreamed possible, meet exciting new people, acquire poise, and learn to make the most of your personality. Travel, glamour, fame, and fortune are all a part of the picture — to a greater or lesser degree, depending on just how much you want to put into modeling. You can model part-time or full-time, earn extra pocket money or fabulous fees, or you can use your modeling as a stepping stone to another career such as acting or designing. You might even, eventually, own your own agency or school, as I do.

1

I have modeled for more fashion designers than I can remember. A sampling would include Dior, Balenciaga, Chanel, Irene, Wragge, Trigère, Rentner, Adrian, and Georgia Bullock. Though I've worked in all phases of modeling, my activities have been mostly in the fashion end of it. Most of my modeling has been in shows—trunk showings and special fashion shows. Fifteen or twenty years ago, my particular figure and size were very much in demand. Sample clothes were made on my type of figure. I was a size 8 or 10; 5 feet 9½ inches tall; had a very small rib cage; a 34-inch bust, 25-inch waist, 35½- to 36-inch hip. This was ideal for many of our top designers then.

Today, the designer's model is shorter and slightly smaller. Although the taller girl still models, she is not as much in demand as she was in my prime. It has been a thrill working for top fashion designers—European and American—in retail shops in New York, California, and Nevada. It was my good fortune to be selected as the right type and size for various designers who featured their styles in particular salons. Any of the designers who wanted a tall model would find me available. I was one of many.

Of course, when I came to live in Las Vegas, my work was done in my own area. It isn't considered a prime area such as New York, Los Angeles, San Francisco, Dallas, or Chicago, but we shouldn't underestimate our own communities. Every community has its own specialty shops who want their clothes modeled by a professional type of girl. A girl can be important in her home area, and she doesn't need to travel to New York or another major area unless she really wants to. She can make money in her own community and enjoy a normal home life along with it.

Many of our busiest models are married and have children. There is an interim period where families will take complete precedence, then back to part-time or full-time modeling. This goes on in any city and from one state to another.

For my readers, I recommend a finishing-school course to teach you the extra poise and polish you will need. It's a great advantage to have someone who is a professional look at you, someone who understands every type of girl and can encourage her along any line. This is not primarily a charm book. Read the book thoroughly once, just for fun, and then go on to study the techniques and the beauty tips. You will find yourself on the way to an exciting world.

I opened the Lenz Finishing and Modeling School in 1960. My purpose in opening it was to bring training and information to girls and women in Las Vegas who had requested my services. We have enlarged it four times since that year, and have become an agency as well. It is now the Lenz Finishing School and Professional Model Agency. Though it has since mushroomed into the largest such school and agency in Nevada, I continually keep studying to keep it the top in its field. I make it my business to take occasional lessons from experts in voice, hair styling, figure control, makeup, and new modeling techniques. It keeps me on the move, too, as I travel to Los Angeles and San Francisco yearly to do this. Being second vice president of the Modeling Association of America takes me regularly to New York, where I brush up on what's new there. There is always something new to learn.

Turning to more practical matters, though, first off you'll probably want to know how much money you can make at modeling.

HOW MUCH CAN YOU EARN?

Money may not actually make the world go around, but it certainly greases the mechanism, so let's talk about the money you can make as a model. Fees will vary for different types of assignments and, even with the same types, will vary from city to city. Let me say right here that, whatever the assignment, a model is well worth her fee. It's only too bad that the fee isn't more standard in each area. Since the wage scale will vary, the average fees I'm giving you here are based on the latest figures available at press time. They will, no doubt, keep changing, but this is a general scale and should give you some idea.

There are extremes between the yearly salary of a top model and what a girl ordinarily will earn as a wholesale or retail model. A top fashion model will earn $30 to $60 an hour. Working throughout the year, she can earn from $50,000 to $100,000. Most models, though, don't work the full twelve months; they either take long vacations or go to Europe to model the coming season's fashion collections. A more likely yearly salary estimate would be somewhere around $15,000 to $20,000.

Photographic Modeling

There is a great deal of money to be made in photographic modeling, and most models will seldom leave it for any other area in the field. Rates are highest in New York and Los Angeles, ranging from $25 to $45 an hour, with a few high-demand models receiving $60 or more. Miami, Detroit, and San Francisco are next, with fees from $25 to $40 an hour. In Las Vegas it's $15 to $30, as it is in Denver and Dallas. Lowest rates seem to apply in the Southeast, with $10 to $20 for Atlanta, $10 to $25 for Louisville, and $10 to $20 for Norfolk, Virginia. Remember, these are average fees. Individual photographers in each city may pay more or less.

Full-Time Modeling

Girls who do wholesale modeling in New York showrooms generally receive weekly salaries that range from $90 to $150. In the smaller garment districts in other cities, models will earn between $60 and $100. Full-time models in retail stores can earn from $90 to $125 in New York, and from $60 to $100 in other areas. In some retail stores, a model may receive a small commission on garments which she shows and sells.

Tearoom Modeling

Tearoom modeling jobs are the "in-between" type, steady work, but not full-time. Many models prefer these jobs so that they can work in other phases of the field.

Department stores or specialty shops have tearoom (luncheon) showings daily or several days a week, and they like to use the same group of models so that customers can identify the models with the store. Fees range from $3.50 to $10 an hour, and the showing usually lasts from one to two hours. At stores paying less, the minimum for a tearoom showing is around $10. As there are no rehearsals, there are no rehearsal fees.

Retail Modeling

These showings are far more lucrative than either tearoom or wholesale modeling. Naturally, they attract the top models, who are the ones hired. In New York salons—department stores or specialty shops—models will earn from $30 to $60 an hour. Fittings are at one-half the model's standard rate.

Los Angeles, San Francisco, Chicago, and Miami pay between $20 and $40 an hour, with fittings and rehearsals at half rates. Fees are lower in the South and Midwest, with department stores paying $15 to $30 per show. In some southeastern cities, the rate goes down to $12.50 per show.

Television Modeling

A television model can make a fortune by working in just one commercial! Not because of her basic earnings, but because of that magic word "residuals." Her basic pay for the bit might bring her $61.50 —including three hours of rehearsal—but she'll receive additional payments *every* time the film is shown. These payments are called "residuals," and I go into them more thoroughly in Chapter 8.

Promotional Modeling

This is another area where the rates vary widely. Promotional modeling can pay as much as $200 a day—for a top model in New York—and as little as $10 for a half day. It depends on where you are, what you're doing, and what you're wearing. This, too, we go into detail in Chapter 8.

That about covers it, as far as your potential earnings are concerned. If you have the face and figure for modeling—and are willing to work hard to achieve that end—you can go right up to the highest bracket. Otherwise, be realistic and choose the field for which you feel you are best suited, and work toward that end. Get an expert opinion on this, too.

TRAVEL IS A FRINGE BENEFIT

Do you like to travel? There's plenty of opportunity for this in the modeling field. I don't mean just traveling to another city to work there, but going out on location assignments. See the world—or the U.S.A.—and get paid for it!

Practically all the magazines that regularly feature fashion—and some that do only a one-shot once in a while—will take a group of models out on location from time to time. *Vogue* and *Harper's Bazaar*, of course, take their models out of the country as unconcernedly as some magazines take them into the next·borough. *Seventeen, Mademoiselle*, and *Glamour* take models out to such places as Honolulu and Acapulco. Europe is practically across the street, and a safari in Africa has been done, too. A fashion safari, naturally!

Not only magazines but cosmetic companies and hair-product firms will take models for location shots out of the state or even out of the country.

Occasionally, too, a designer will take a collection—and his models—out of the country, like the group of fashion models who went to Russia in 1967 for a special showing behind the Iron Curtain. That's *really* seeing the world!

YOU'LL MEET NEW PEOPLE

By its very nature, showing clothes and thereby selling them, modeling is a means of meeting people. You work with designers, fashion coordinators, makeup artists, and hair stylists, and you're showing to customers, buyers, the press, and many other persons. You meet people both ways.

At conventions and when you're doing any kind of promotional modeling, you'll meet hundreds of people in any one day. You're required to make contact and get a message across to them. If you never see any one of these people again in your life, you're still getting valuable experience for your future contacts with people in your personal life. It will do wonders for your poise, and make you a person everyone will enjoy being with.

THE FUN OF WORKING WITH CLOTHES

Is there any woman alive who doesn't love clothes? From the ancient days, when elegant Egyptian ladies changed from simple, straight, ankle-length sheaths to fine accordion-pleated overskirts, fashion has been a favorite subject for women of all ages. They find a keen delight in exploring every facet of fashion — seeing, touching, discussing, buying, and wearing.

On the other side of the coin, you'll find the people who actually work to bring us the new styles we so admire with a view to wearing them. Many of the designers, as well as owners of salons, are men, but there is still one area of the fashion world where the female of the species reigns supreme — and that is in the showing of the new designs. Here is where the fashion model has it all her own way and is really in her glory.

If you love wearing clothes, think how much more thrilling it will be for you to have a part in bringing new ideas to other women! You can be an important part of a fascinating world, whether you're a high-priced salon model showing one-of-a-kind originals to a wealthy clientele, or modeling in your own community for the town's only dress shop. You will find as much satisfaction either way, and you'll be wearing beautiful new styles and getting paid for it. In fact, you can have just as much fun if you aren't getting paid and are modeling for a charity fashion show in your area. You'll find a whole section on putting on your own fashion show in my last chapter, and once you've done one for your organization you may never go back again to bridge games to raise money.

Whichever aspect of modeling you decide upon, the end result is the same. You'll have the absolute joy of working with new fashions. You'll learn to know fabrics, designers' styles, lines, everything that goes to make a costume a little bit different from any other. Even if you never earn a penny from modeling, you'll be able to apply all you've learned to your own wardrobe, and you may easily wind up as the best-dressed woman in your town. And you'll have the complete satisfaction of feeling and looking like a model.

THE THRILL OF IT ALL

While we're so busy being practical and sensible about the field, let's not lose sight of the fact that modeling, after all, is a glamorous profession. The very word "model" conjures up visions of sequins and champagne, dancing until dawn, and dozens of dashing escorts. This is seldom literally true, but the picture itself is seductive enough.

Yes, there is glamour in modeling and it's to be found in every phase. It is, however, a matter of degree. I personally think the whole field has a glamour about it. Taking the literal meaning of the word "glamour," which is "enchantment" or "a magic spell," you can apply it to any aspect of modeling. Of course you're casting a spell when you can take a scrap of silk or velvet, or any fabric, and bring it to life just by showing it in a special way, wearing it in a special manner. An entire fashion show — if it's well staged and presented — is really only weaving a gigantic enchantment, and you are the star bringing to life all the femininity the designs demand.

Proceeding from the overall glamour to the individual kind, it's up to you and your qualifications. While this book is definitely dedicated to the principle that *anyone* can model — and that means the ordinarily attractive, reasonably intelligent female in any age group in any community — this doesn't exclude those among you who have unusual beauty or that certain aura that makes a great model. Who's to say that you won't be next year's Jean Shrimpton, or Wilhelmina, or — if you're young enough and thin enough — next year's version of Twiggy!

If you make it, the world will truly be your oyster. You'll see yourself smiling from magazine covers, be invited to all the gala openings, be asked to endorse products, write books, head cosmetic lines. You'll have all the trappings and privileges of a superstar for as long as you care and work to keep them.

You might even marry a famous designer or owner of a fashion house, which is not unheard of, though unlikely, because there aren't that many designers to go around. Pretty, green-eyed Maryll Lanvin, the wife of the heir to the famous house of Lanvin, is the star model who opens the show at each major collection and is a source of inspiration to house designer Jules François Crahay. You can hardly become more glamorous than that!

A STEPPING STONE TO ANOTHER CAREER

Modeling can serve you well in two ways—or more—depending on how ambitious you are and where your other talents lie. The things you learn in modeling can stand you in good stead if you decide to pursue other lines of work.

Your basic techniques—posture, walking, projecting, etc.—can form an excellent background to an acting career. Famous models who went into acting include Suzy Parker and Charlene Holt, France's Capucine, and England's Glenna Forster-Jones. Grace Kelly was a top Ford model and now she reigns as a princess. Lucille Ball was a model for designer Hattie Carnegie. Barbara Feldon, the star of NBC-TV's "Get Smart," was formerly the Revlon "Tiger" girl, and before that, she claims, she was an overweight housewife. *That* should be encouraging.

Do you want to be a writer? The world of fashion is fascinating enough to give you material for all kinds of writing, if you have a way with a word. Jean Shrimpton, Anita Colby, and Twiggy are models who have written books.

Sometimes you can combine more than one career with your modeling, or as a result of it. Jean Shrimpton—known affectionately as "The Shrimp"—is the head of a line of hair-care products for Yardley of London. Twiggy lends her name to a line of eye makeup for the same company. Anita Colby is a commentator for fashion shows and TV. Candy Jones has a charm school. Jinx Falkenburg has had her own TV show and does occasional TV commentating chores. Betty Furness was one of the original stars of TV commercials, and Wilhelmina has her own model agency. I have my own school and agency, am a fashion commentator, do TV, and have written a book. In my case, at any rate, one thing inevitably seems to follow another.

So use your modeling know-how as a springboard to other things. Learn all you can and apply all you learn to areas that are closely allied. It means doing more than exactly what you're called upon to do. It means research and extra study, but ultimately you will be equipped to take on much more than you originally intended. Then, who knows how far you can go? Today a model—tomorrow the world!

2
MODEL TYPES AND FIGURES

Modeling is for everyone. There is a need for every age, size, figure, and type. With so many categories within the medium itself, any girl with the proper qualifications and attitudes—and the proper training—should be able to find a suitable spot for herself somewhere within the field.

All models aren't glamorous and exotic, or even necessarily beautiful. Just look at the plain Jane doing a detergent commercial, and realize that this girl is a model too. She does commercial modeling. The requirements are different, but it's still one of the many facets of a fascinating profession. You may not be the type to do fashion modeling, but you could be exactly right for commercials. Of course, you'd need some extras such as a knowledge of acting, but your basic training in modeling techniques and personality development will form an invaluable background for this, as well as for every other, phase of the business.

So many different types are needed. The wholesome girl is as much in demand as the exquisite "cover" girl. She'll be in a different category, but she'll be used. When you come right down to it, even the radiant fashion models aren't all flawlessly beautiful, but they've learned the art of making it appear that way.

You don't realize it, but when you pick up a copy of *Vogue* or *Harper's Bazaar*, you're really looking at the top photographic models in the business. They're beautiful and exotic, and they're literally at the top of the ladder. But what about the thousands of other models who work on New York's Seventh Avenue and in the various wholesale houses and department stores all over the country? They all have one thing in common with the girls in the fashion magazines. They have a particular *look*. Each girl looks and acts like a model. So can you. Find your place, and then fill it brilliantly.

9

The four major classifications in modeling are:

I.   Fashion Modeling—wholesale, retail, salon, tearoom.
II. Photographic Modeling—magazines, newspapers.
III. Television and Motion Picture Modeling.
IV. Promotional Modeling—exhibits, conventions.

You can prepare for any of these by learning the techniques, whether you go into the commercial or the fashion end. You may start with one aspect of the craft, and then go into another. You never really know until you're actually in the field. The important thing is that you *can* model somewhere. I will go into detail about the various types of modeling in a later chapter, and you can find out where your particular type would shine best. Right now, let's concentrate on individual types.

AGES AND SIZES

I will explain each category in detail, but here are your age and size groups at a glance:

1. Little Miss—five to ten years.
2. Little Miss Pre-Teen—eleven to twelve years.
3. Junior Miss—thirteen to seventeen years.
4. Collegiate—seventeen to twenty-two years—5 feet 5 inches to 5 feet 9 inches in height. (This is a look, not a size. The model need not be in this age group).
5. High Fashion—eighteen to thirty-five years—5 feet 7 inches to 5 feet 9½ inches.
6. Junior Petite and Petite—any age over thirteen—5 feet 2 inches to 5 feet 6 inches in height.
7. Half Size—usually over thirty years—wears a half size, 12½ to 18½ and up.
8. Senior Sophisticate—over forty years—5 feet 6 inches to 5 feet 9½ inches.

Children

1. Babies to four-and-one-half years
2. Little Miss, five to ten years
3. Little Miss, Pre-Teens

Every age is used. Babies are needed for commercials, but require no direction. When we get into the actual fashion field—which is what we're discussing now—the correct way of doing things is a must. In fashion-show modeling, the little two-year-old girl who clings so charmingly to her mother's or a model's hand needs no training, but I would say that a good age for a professional child model is from five to ten. Each age as well as each year has its own category, but the average child model may start her training from five to ten and on up to the teens.

The Pre-Teen is in a category of her own. She'd be about eleven or twelve years old, possibly thirteen. It depends on how old she looks and what size she wears. Little children ranging from five on would be wearing sizes 4 to 6X. As they grow older, they'll go into the slightly larger sizes—7's and 8's, 9's and 10's. It all depends on what the store or the manufacturer wants to show in size ranges. They're the ones who decide on the types and sizes needed.

Usually a fashion show that wants to cover all age brackets will show a five-year-old, a ten-year-old, a Pre-Teen or thirteen-year-old, and then go into the fourteen- to fifteen- and sixteen- to seventeen-year span. Every age is needed. In general, it would seem a model would have to be within a twenty- to twenty-five-age limit, but when we come right down to essentials, clothes are made for every age and every type of figure. Everyone wants to imagine herself having the perfect figure, so consequently you will rarely see a full figure in a fashion show, unless the manufacturer or store is specifically showing larger-size clothes. The ideal in a fashion show is definitely a slim, trim figure—at any age.

Junior Miss, Junior Petite, and Petite

Now we go into the Junior and Petite sizes, which are 5, 7, 8, 9, and 12. Junior Petite is cut for a shorter figure. For example, a typical weekly fashion show that tries to cover all ages—I do two or more of these a week that will include a child—will have one who wears a 5 to 6X one week. Next week there will be a child wearing 8 to 10. In the same show we'll have a petite girl (about 5 feet 1 inch) who wears a Junior Petite 5 or 7. Then we'll go into a Junior Miss in a 5 or 7. The difference is that the Junior Miss is cut for a less mature figure and for a younger girl. She may be short-to-average height, and she's smaller bosomed. She would be about 5 feet 2 inches to 5 feet 5 inches in height.

When you get into Petites for adults, it's an entirely different cut, and the manufacturer will select a woman or a Young Sophisticate model who's 5 feet 4 inches or under. Usually the height will range from 5 feet 2 inches to 5 feet 4 inches. A girl under 5 feet 5 inches is in between. She can wear some Petites and some regular 7's or 8's. It all depends on the structure of her body.

With an all-adult show, we can still show Petite, regular, and fuller figure sizes. Petites would be 5 feet 4 inches and under in height, and the sizes are 5, 6, 7, and 8. These will vary with the individual

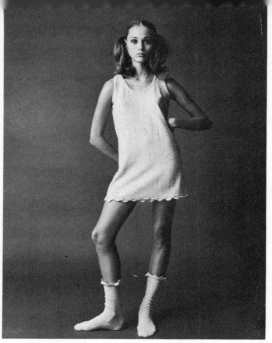

Jane Hitchcock of Wilhelmina Model Agency, wears sizes 5, 6, 7. A darling Junior Miss type.

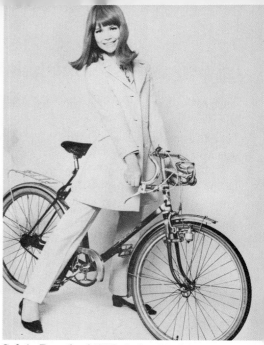

Sylvia Poorth of Wilhelmina Model Agency is capable of looking very collegiate, as you see here. Sylvia, with a change of hairpieces and expression, can also appear very High Fashion. Wears sizes 5, 7, 9, is 5 feet 7½ inches tall.

girl, of course. I have several models who are 5 feet 4½ inches tall and wear size 8 beautifully.

The model who is considered the ideal height today would be 5 feet 7 inches to 5 feet 8½ inches tall, and she would wear size 8 or 10. This is the average model. She is more in demand, but Petites are needed and are becoming quite prominent in fashion. More and more houses are designing for Petites, aware that there are more small than tall women.

High Fashion—Young Sophisticates (the Twenties)

There are so many fine shadings regarding the different types of models that often the categories overlap. But who is used the most? It's the girl who is 5 feet 7 inches to 5 feet 8½ inches and who wears a size 8 or 10. The girl who works the most will look—she may not be that age, but she will look—between twenty-one and twenty-six. This is her prime time as far as the Sophisticate goes. Otherwise she is definitely in one of the other categories we're discussing. She may be a Collegiate type in one photograph, High Fashion in another.

High Fashion—Sophisticate (the Thirties)

The prime years of modeling probably would be from nineteen to twenty-nine. After that, it depends on how you hold your looks.

I have girls who are thirty-five and look only twenty-eight or twenty-nine. In fact, there are many models all over the country who are in their mid-thirties and still look as if they were in their mid-twenties. There are models who have worked for the same photographer for over a decade and are still very much in demand for the same age group in which they started out, and a camera is much more exacting. It's all in the way a girl cares for herself. (See "Tearoom Modeling," Chapter 8.)

Half Size

Manufacturers of Half-Size clothes use a model who is fuller in the figure and slightly shorter in the waist than the regular model. She may range from 5 feet 4 inches to 5 feet 7½ inches in height. In fashion shows, she would wear size 12½ to 16½. However, Half-Size clothes can be purchased to 24½. Needless to say, this is not the best Half-Size to feature in a fashion show. In most cases, the model used will be a mature woman rather than a young model under twenty-five years of age.

Senior Sophisticate (the Forties, Fifties, and Older)

The matronly model—we like to call her the smart matron or Senior Sophisticate—is not used too frequently in New York, although you will see her in the catalogs. At New York fashion shows, however,

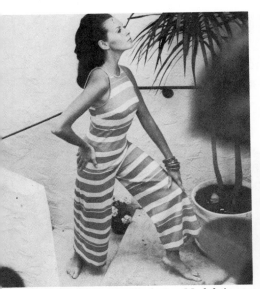

Mary Madden of Wilhelmina Model Agency is another versatile model. Wears sizes 8, 10, 12, is 5 feet 8½ inches tall. Good bone structure such as Mary possesses photographs well.

Photo by John Haynesworth

Bernie Lenz (left) presents first-place award trophy to lovely silver-haired Lenz model Dorothy Uhouse. Dorothy modeled in the Senior Sophisticate Model competition in the Waldorf Astoria Hotel during the Modeling Association of America Convention, 1968. She is 5 feet 6 inches tall, size 12. There is definitely a place for our models past forty.

Photo by Drucker-Hilbert

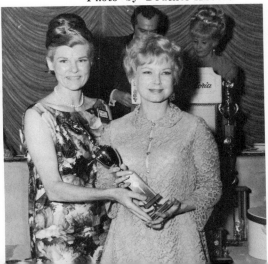

she is thoroughly missed. Happily enough, this is not the case in the majority of fashion shows in other cities throughout the country.

This is the way it should be. After all, most of the women who have money to buy clothes are past thirty, forty, or fifty years of age. They want to see what they'll like in the new designs, so there's a definite field for the Senior Sophisticate. It's growing rapidly, because a woman wants to see a real, human being in her own age group. Not an ideally young, divinely willowy, and absolutely perfect creature who bears little or no resemblance to herself!

The Senior Sophisticate, of course, should have a good figure. She can be slightly rounded in a matronly way, but she still must be able to wear a size 10 or 12. With a petite woman, the height would be 5 feet 4 inches again, and you'd also have your average and tall Senior Sophisticate model. The tall one may be a size 12 or 14. With any sizes beyond that, you simply won't have as smart a woman. Occasionally she may be a size 16, but ideally she should be a flexible 12 or 14, and possibly be able to wear a size 16, if necessary.

As long as she stays within these size limits and keeps her figure proportionately bal nced, the Senior Sophisticate certainly has her place. I hope that many of our smart-looking matronly women will learn from this book and enjoy the field of modeling. I've trained many women who originally thought they were going to spend the rest of their lives sitting at home, with nothing inspiring to look forward to once the children were raised and gone. They were quite surprised when I told them, "You would make a nice model, so let's train you and use you in some fashion shows."

And invariably your Senior Sophisticate model will steal the show! It's either the five-year-old model or the Senior Sophisticate. These are the two types that receive the most applause. We all know a child will rate applause, but why the matron? Well, she receives the ovation because one does admire a handsomely dressed woman over forty. When I say "matron," I am referring to a woman past forty. She's sophisticated, she's smart, her figure is excellent, and she carries herself superbly. Elegant as she is, however, she is past forty and so must go into the matron category — or, more appropriately, Senior Sophisticate — and be able to enjoy every minute of it.

This is why modeling can be such a joy throughout an entire lifetime. There are youngsters who started in modeling at five, and every five years — or every two years — changed sufficiently to become a different type of model. Once a girl reaches eighteen, she becomes the Young Sophisticate model, and then swings into the Sophisticate model when she's in her middle twenties and early thirties.

Then she will find that every ten years will mark a change. At thirty, she will model differently than she did when she was twenty, at forty, differently than when she was thirty, and at fifty, she will model in still another way. She will carry just a hint of a different air about her, always smart and chic, but there is a change. And from fifty to sixty, it is just a little bit different. Yet she should remain aware of *not being old.*

"Old" is not a term we should ever use lightly. No one is ever really old. You've simply reached a different plateau, and you still should be constantly aware of looking smart. As for the lucky woman who can manage to do this for extra part-time or full-time work as a model, she will be much more on her toes—and proudly so—in keeping up with the new trends.

I can't put this too strongly. I certainly want to encourage our older women to become aware of their potential. This is the time and these are the years when you should want to take yourselves in hand and take care of your figure, your posture, and your general well-being. I know it takes effort. It's so easy to just slide back and let your figure go. Don't let it happen.

Make the most of yourself. Learn to model, learn to give a fashion show, make money for your organization, and have a marvelous time doing it. You can learn to become an integral part of a whole magical new world, and your entire life will be brightened by it.

GENERAL PHYSICAL QUALIFICATIONS

Measurements

Basically, the average model should be between 5 feet 6 inches and 5 feet 9 inches in height. Her bust should measure 34 inches, her waist 24 to 26 inches, and her hips should be between 35 and 37 inches. These measurements would be proportionately larger if a model is taller. The ideal hip measurement would be 35 inches, but once in a while your 5 feet 9 inch- or 5 feet 10 inch-girl might have a 37-inch hip and wear a size 10. This, again, is determined by a girl's individual body structure, but 35 to 36 inches for hips are average. Her measurements from the back are important, and whether she is short-waisted or long-waisted. If a girl is too short- or long-waisted, this may handicap her. She should be able to wear average cuts in clothes and, if she has to err in any direction at all, she should be a bit long-waisted for high fashion.

As for a model's body build, it is a must that she be not too bosomy, at least at the present stage of fashion. Later on, who knows? Right now, though, most fashion models would be average to small. Some girls, of course, are very clever about buying bras. Always buy bras that are rounded and natural; then you can adjust them if necessary. No padding, except certain little extras I'll tell you about when we discuss "A Model's Bag of Tricks." There are various ingenious ways of rounding out a contour if you have to fit a special garment you're planning to model.

The ideal model should have a nice, trim waistline — this goes without saying, but we'll make sure and say it! — and a small, neat rib cage. We are naturally assuming she doesn't have any surplus fat around the waistline, or anywhere else. Hips should be nicely fashioned, with just enough subtle curvature. She should have perfect posture, not be swaybacked or have the appearance of too big a derriere. The derriere can be slightly rounded, but, in any case, a slim fashion model, because of weight reduction and keeping her weight down, will not have too much of a derriere. After all, every girl is shaped differently. If, however, a girl is too flat in the back, never mind. There are many clever tricks in the trade that work wonders. We'll discuss them later on.

Legs

A model's legs are so important that they almost deserve a whole chapter for themselves. A girl *must* have beautiful legs if she's going to be truly successful, though I have seen models who have done very well in the fashion field in spite of having legs that were not as slim as they would wish. They make up for the slight lack by keeping their weight down and having nicely shaped legs as well as by being extra special models in other ways. So, just because a girl doesn't have a really thin shapely leg doesn't mean she won't be able to model.

This would be a must in New York, where standards are so exacting. This, after all, is where much of the photographic modeling is done, and these are the models who are seen all over the country and the world. Standards for them are more exacting than for the girls who work in wholesale or retail.

In other locales, a girl can have a satisfying successful career if she is a lovely model in every other way. I have two or three models of this type. They don't actually have heavy legs, but they aren't as slim as they would like them to be. Yet these girls are excellent models, and they have done — and are doing — beautifully in the profession.

I emphasize what New York wants in a model, because there they want as close to perfection as possible. The field there is much more critical, but there are many average-size towns where a girl can have success in fashion modeling without being perfect. If she knows how to model smoothly, carry herself beautifully, and excel in every other way, she can still make money modeling.

Bone Structure

A good model will be either small- or average-boned. Again, though, I have seen large-boned girls lose weight, keep their figures trim and slim, and be terrific models. This would not go in New York, as you can suppose. She must be small-boned in New York. Sometimes, however, an average-boned girl can keep her weight down and actually appear small-boned. It's worth keeping in mind.

Facial Features

Requirements here vary for photographic and fashion modeling. A fashion model doesn't have to be the beautiful "All-American Girl" type, but she should have well-spaced eyes and a nose that isn't too broad. She may have a slightly longer nose—it can actually be an asset to her—and with proper shading and a skillful makeup, she can have an interesting look. She could even have a bump on her nose, if it's properly camouflaged. She does her work onstage, so it isn't as critical as if she were facing a camera. An average-to-full mouth will be more advantageous, as well as a lovely smile and good teeth.

Teeth need not be perfect for stage work because, again, the model is seen only by the naked eye and not by the merciless all-seeing eye of a camera. After all, you don't normally walk around smiling and showing your teeth, so a good model will learn how to smile without exposing her teeth. If you have a fairly nice set of teeth, you generally can manage very well in fashion modeling.

If you have any obviously crooked or ugly teeth—and these are the only imperfections you have that might keep you from successful modeling—I think it would be a profitable investment to have the offenders capped or straightened. See your orthodontist and have him analyze your problem. Then follow through and have it solved.

A slim face is good, and high cheekbones are most desirable. On the other hand, there are many square faces with such basically good bone structure that the only thing needed to bring out the high cheekbones is a loss of weight. Even with a round face, if one has high cheekbones, a suitable loss of weight will emphasize them. A model should have a shapely and well-proportioned chin. A generally good bone structure will take care of this, too.

A too-round or too-short neck is not good. An average-to-longer neck would be an important asset and, in the high-fashion field, the slightly longer neck would be better.

HOW LONG CAN YOU GO ON MODELING?

We've covered ages, sizes, types, and general physical qualifications. Now for the big question. How long can you go on modeling? The answer is—as long as you like! It's all in the way you take care of yourself.

Be scrupulous about keeping your figure trim, your skin flawless, and yourself supple. Keeping a youthful skin, incidentally, doesn't only depend on good care and proper cleansing. These are most important, but you must learn—when you're young—not to squint, frown, tug at your underlip, or pull at the skin underneath your chin. These mannerisms and habits are probably unconscious, but do try to keep aware of them and when you catch yourself indulging—stop!

The less you grimace, the fewer wrinkles you'll have to worry about. Of course, don't be drastic and stop smiling or laughing altogether! These activities may eventually end up in extra lines, too, but it takes much longer, and lines created this way aren't nearly as unattractive as the others.

So, if she is careful, a girl can extend her years of modeling sophisticated fashions almost indefinitely. And when she finally has to move on to the next category, she can do so gracefully and with a flourish.

3
LEARNING TECHNIQUES

Now that you know something about the modeling profession, the types of models needed, and the many advantages connected with the field, you're ready to learn the basic techniques. This is a most important chapter. I'd suggest you read it straight through once, at first. Read it casually, just to allow it to make a preliminary impression and give you the feel of things. Then take it section by section. Learn each movement or attitude, practice it, and try to have it as perfect as possible before you go on to the next.

The only props you'll need will be a full-length mirror and a record player or a radio. If you have a sympathetic but objective girl friend you can press into service, fine. Later on, if you like, you can expand your audience to include your family and more of your friends.

All of these movements and positions will be new to the aspiring model, but there are many professionals who—knowing many of the techniques—will still be able to use the instructions as a convenient brush-up to keep them on their toes. They pick them up very quickly because they already know the basics. Perhaps they may perceive—and so correct—faulty areas that they've been unaware of until now. Many girls who have studied modeling want to know more, and this can be their way of learning more.

So, beginners and professionals alike, get out the mirror, turn on the music whenever you're ready, *and get to work!*

A MODEL'S POSTURE

A model's posture is the beginning. It is the most important requisite throughout her career. She must carry herself like a queen. Re-

19

member, a model's objective is to show off clothes to the very best advantage. If a model has poor posture, she doesn't get the first job. So let's work on that posture. We'll start out with an exercise which, at the same time, will show you how you'll be lining up your body properly. Follow the photographs carefully. You'll notice that our model is wearing a leotard, so that you'll learn more by seeing the whole body.

1. Stand up against the wall, feet together, letting your heels, your derriere, your shoulders, and your head touch the wall. Pull up your rib cage, tuck buttocks under, and flex the knees. If you can put a full hand between the wall and your waist, you are not sufficiently tucked under. You have—to put it bluntly—a swayback.

2. *Exercise for Swayback*—With your back against the wall, your feet together and about 10 inches away from the baseboard, relax your arms. Bend forward slowly from the waist, head down. While in this position make a conscious effort to push the spine upward by stretching each vertebra. After stretching the spine, come up slowly, head still down, starting with the waist, and press each vertebra against the wall until your head touches. Then, lean over again and repeat this ten times. Go down to your sitting position.

1. Stand up against wall.

2. Swayback exercise. Bend over and roll-spin from waist to head.

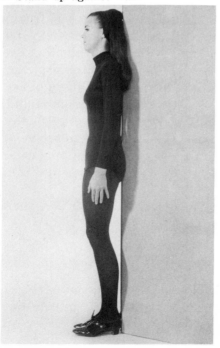

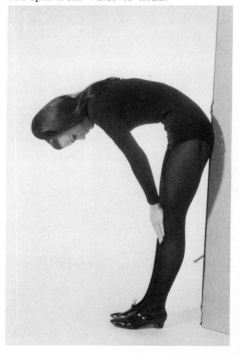

3. From the standing position, bend your knees slowly, pressing your body down the wall to a sitting position. Your spine should flatten against the wall so no one can put a hand between the wall and it. Hold the position for a count of 6. By holding the tummy muscles very tight at this point, you are also doing a fine isometric exercise to help your swayback and tighten your tummy muscles.

If you're very swaybacked, it would probably be wise to start with your feet about 10 inches away from the wall and — with your head, shoulders, and derriere touching the wall — try to flatten your spine as you go into the sitting position again. Hold it for a count of a slow 6 or a fast 10 — whichever you find easier.

4. To check your shoulders and make sure you haven't acquired a dowager's hump — or to correct a dowager's hump — let's take the position of feet together, 10 inches away from the wall, with spine flattened against the wall. Place your fingernails, shoulder high, back up against the wall. Your elbows should be touching the wall. Your head, your shoulders, your elbows, and your derriere are touching — and your spine is flat against — the wall. Remember, your feet are together and about 10 inches away from the baseboard. Slowly, but in one continuous movement, raise your arms above your head . . .

3. Swayback and upper thigh exercise combination. Hold for six counts.

4. Flatten spine to wall, place fingernails and elbows shoulder high.

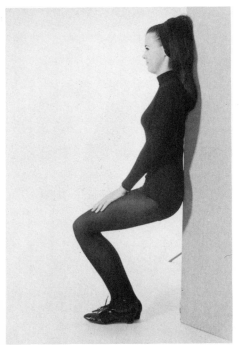

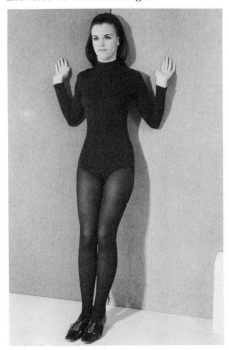

5. . . . keeping your nails and elbows touching the wall. You will probably feel a strain through the upper shoulders near the neck, where a dowager's hump would be apt to develop. Now bring fingernails, elbows, hands, and arms back to shoulder level again. Do this ten times daily if you have any tendency to a dowager's hump or a forward-thrust head. This is particularly good for the shoulders; if there is any roundness in there, it will work itself out. Keep that spine close to the wall, and tuck under.

You cannot correct a poor posture by simply *thinking* posture. You must exercise and loosen those muscles to get them working properly. You must check your posture a half-dozen times a day.

How do you check your posture? By "walking" up to the wall and lining yourself up with the wall.

6. Your ears should be lined up with your shoulders, your arms with your knees, and your fingertips should be hanging straight down the side seam of your dress. Back up against the wall, so that the back of your head, back of your shoulders, your derriere, and your heels are touching it. Is it comfortable? Are you tucked under? Can you barely get four fingers between the wall and the small of your back? You shouldn't be able to push a full hand through—just the four fingers. The knees are always flexed.

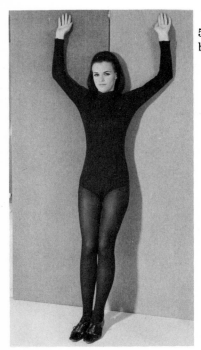

6. Can you draw a straight line from your ears, shoulders, fingertips, knees, and weight on the balls of your feet?

5. Raise hands high above head and lower back to shoulder height. Repeat ten times.

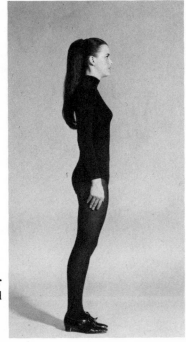

A most important element of a model's posture is the way she carries her head and holds her neck. There should be an awareness of the head held high. Feel that you are pushing the top of your head to the ceiling. This is vital to a queenly look. Your chin should look as if it is sitting on a shelf—I know this sounds funny—and be parallel to the floor. You should actually feel that you're trying to stretch your neck back of the ears right out of your shoulders. If you are inclined to have a short neck, or one that's perhaps a little bit thick, you can make it appear longer or thinner by stretching your chin and your neck until you feel tightness, and then holding it for a count of 6. It is essential to pull the neck up out of the shoulders. Don't allow it to sink into them. This is vital to a beautiful carriage.

One more word about posture. If you have a very bad posture, I am not beyond saying that you should try a shoulder brace. You can buy one in any good surgical supply store, or through a surgical supply catalog. Buy a brace and wear it. It's a marvelous reminder. Start out by using it four hours a day. It can really work wonders.

You know how to get—and keep—correct posture now. You'll have to learn to adjust to the wishes of the designer when it comes to specific instances. Just remember that a designer may ask you to take a slightly different posture. Adjust to his needs. Just walk out tall and relaxed. Let's smile!

A MODEL'S STANCE

I'd like you to stand tall, place your feet together, face straight into a mirror, and look at your legs. Do the calves meet? Do the knees and upper thighs touch? Since most models are slim, chances are that their legs will not meet somewhere along the line. The model's stance will eliminate any imperfection, as it gives a slight angle to the body, which is why a model uses it. We also assume various different foot positions from this basic stance.

1, 2. Standing up and facing the mirror, place your heels together and point your toes out at a 45-degree angle, in a ballet position. Let's leave the weight on the right foot, pick up the left, bring it around to the front, and point it straight to the audience. Your left foot now should be pointing straight ahead and the heel should be approximately an inch and a half or two inches away from the right foot, which is the back foot. Looking into the mirror, you should be able to see the heel and toe of the back foot. This is a nice, even model's stance.

Knees are never stiff in modeling; they're always slightly flexed. The front knee should not be bent or completely relaxed, just barely flexed. Of course, later on this would depend on what you're actually modeling. You might find it proper and appropriate to bend your knee at times.

Now you should try this position with your left foot behind you and your right foot pointing. Either way, it's still a model's stance, but it's prettier in this position.

At this point, we can talk about the upstage foot and the downstage foot. The foot *closest* to your audience is called your downstage foot. The foot *farthest* away from the audience is your upstage foot.

Some wag is surely going to make a joke about "What if *both* feet are together?" Then there isn't any special foot — there can't be a downstage or an upstage foot. Both feet are even. Both are downstage, but when one is in front of the other, we have to designate which it is.

Now for Stage Left and Stage Right. When you're facing the audience, if you lift your left arm and point it to your left, that is Stage Left. Take your right arm and point it over to your right — that is Stage Right. These positions remain the same, regardless of what way you're facing.

If you find yourself getting rather confused here, don't give up. It really becomes quite simple in practice. And think how handy this training is going to be if you decide to go on to a dramatic career! These are the same stage directions you would get from your director, though he may vary them sometimes. He may refer to downstage as "walking toward the footlights" or "toward the edge of the stage," and he

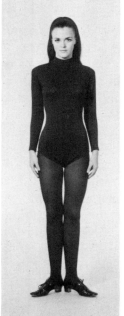

1. Stand with heels together, feet out at 45-degree angle.

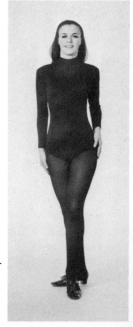

2. Point left foot straight ahead. Approximately 2 inches apart.

may refer to upstage as "toward the back wall" or "toward the curtain," if there is one at the back.

Just keep practicing these stage directions until you find yourself automatically heading the right way. Remember, when you're facing an audience, your *left* is their *right* — and vice versa.

3. You get a prettier effect in a model's stance if your hip is turned back a little to get more of a three-quarter view of the figure. Notice the difference when the body is turned slightly. Keeping the toe pointed to the audience and then bringing the shoulder back, you get more of a silhouette view, and this is important. If you always try to bring about a three-quarter view to your audience, it is a more attractive look.

If a girl is very thin, this isn't too serious, but it does give a prettier line to the body and a silhouette to the bust line.

ASSIGNMENT

    1. Practice model's stance with the right foot behind you.

    2. Practice model's stance with the left foot behind you.

    3. Try your model's stance with the three-quarter view.

    4. Practice your stage directions. Have a friend call out "Stage Right," "Stage Left," "Upstage," "Downstage."

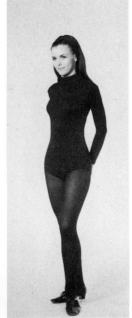

3. Three-quarter view of body more attractive.

A MODEL'S WALK

How to Walk

A model must walk with an airy lightness as well as with a tremendous smoothness. The weight is always forward. The body should never appear stiff.

Now, think and feel that a gentle wind is pushing you along. Your feet are reaching with much the same feeling as if you were walking downhill. The majority of women use the *front* foot for propulsion, whereas a smoother walk is obtained by letting the *back* foot push you into the next step.

Too much emphasis cannot be placed on the importance of letting your back foot push you into the next step—to give that light feeling. You might pretend you're walking on foam rubber, and you can't stop! Or that you're walking on eggs. Anything you can imagine so that your feet will have a feeling of lightness. Reach—reach—reach with your front foot, push with your back foot, and feel that faint breath of a breeze that is propelling you along.

Let's learn from the following illustrations.

1. Correct Side View
    1. Rib cage up and body straight, but not stiff.
    2. Arms down the seams of your dress, palms in.
    3. Shoulders down, back, and relaxed.
    4. Head up, feel your chin is on a shelf.
    5. Tight tuck-under of buttocks, tummy in and firm.
    6. Knees are always flexed.
    7. Steps just long enough to keep body erect.

1. Correct side view.   2. Incorrect side views.

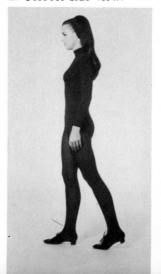
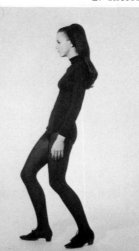
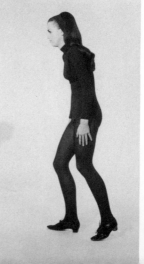

2. Incorrect Side View
    1. Too long steps.
    2. Extreme bend of knees.
    3. Round shoulders.
    4. Sunken rib cage.
    5. Neck forward.

3. Check yourself in a mirror. Avoid showing a space between the legs when walking, and any side hip movement.

4. To check your foot position, draw a straight line on the floor, and place your big toe joint and heel along this line. Step forward about 2 inches, still aligning the heel and toe joint with the line. Look into the mirror and make sure that there is no space showing between your legs. If there is space, close in the heel and foot slightly to correct this open area. Now take another step, letting your knees gently brush each other, and learn the feel of correct placement of legs and feet. Keep looking in the mirror to check your legs. You must feel exactly where your legs are touching so that you will know you are walking correctly when onstage.

5. This is the way you should look when walking. The back foot is pushing you into the correct forward step, and you will glide along beautifully. There should be no hesitation, nor any heavy weight in the heels. Just one long, lovely, and effortless glide.

3. Avoid space between legs.

4. Place big toe joint and heel on a straight line. Make adjustments to close any open space.

5. Reach with the ball of your foot and let that back foot push and glide you along smoothly.

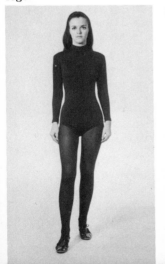
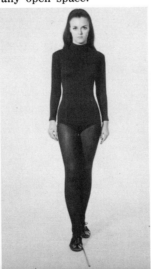
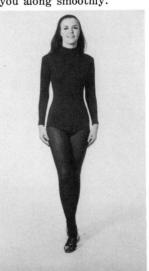

Note: The toe of your shoe will be approximately one inch on the other side of the line. Never align the point of your shoe exactly with the line. You need this slight toe-over-line for balance.

Speed of walk: This should be approximately nine steps in five seconds. Basically, you should not be slow with your walk. However, you must learn to adjust the speed of your walk to the costume, the size of the individual stage, or to the music.

How to Balance

Now and again, a girl has trouble with her balance. This need not be disturbing. A simple exercise will correct the condition. This exercise is actually an exaggeration of normal walking.

1. Bringing one leg up, stand straight. You may start without shoes and then work into wearing shoes with heels.
2. Straighten your leg and bring your foot down in the process of walking. Keep your body straight.
3. Step forward. Heel of back foot raises as toe and heel of front foot touch the floor.
4. Begin to raise other leg. Keep the legs close. Knee up and repeat.

Note: These are highly exaggerated motions of walking, but, basically, walking is just these motions. You bend the knees, straighten them, and reach and push into the next step. This exercise is very good for balancing.

1. Bring one leg up.

2. Straighten leg and point toe down.

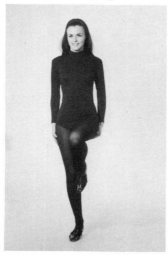

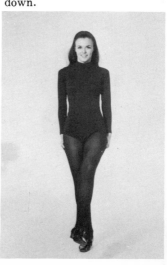

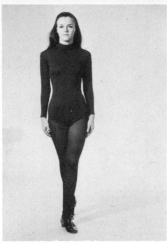

3. Start to bring right knee up with next step.

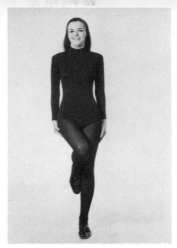

4. Raise the right leg, and repeat.

How to Step and Swing Arms

LENGTH OF STEP

1. Using a chair for a prop, take hold of chair back and rise up on your toes.
2. Put one foot forward and stretch it out.
3. Now bring it straight down, without bending the knees. Where the foot touches the floor will determine the length of your step — half the length of your foot, usually. Please note that the body must be straight. Otherwise it will lean over.

1. Hold onto chair. Up on your toes.

2. Keeping knee straight, bring one foot up off the floor. Point toe.

3. Bring the toe down to touch the floor. Keep the body straight. You will find your front foot will be about 2 inches in front of the back foot.

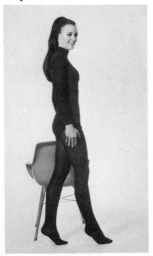

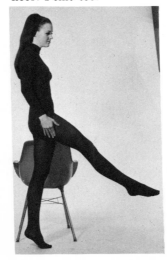

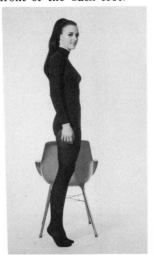

ARM SWING

1, 2. The arms should not detract from the clothes being modeled, therefore they should not swing out more than the width of the body. Keep arms loose and easy, hanging from the shoulders, never bending at the elbows. The thumb can literally touch the costume while keeping it in that close.

Note: Facing your full-length mirror, practice your arm swings and check the length of your step.

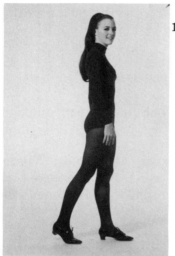

1. Swing width of body.

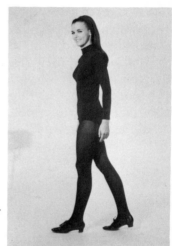

2. Swing width of body, thumbs gently brushing garment.

MODEL TURNS

Model's Half Turn

The Half Turn will be used in combination with other pivots, but it is the first step in learning to turn on the balls of your feet. Practice your Half Turns carefully until you achieve the smooth, graceful, *continuous* motion that is so important.

Imagine your mirror is your audience. Stand in front of it in a model's stance (see above); you should have your weight going down through the center of your body and into the balls of your feet. You should feel no weight in your heels. Both knees are flexed. Follow the illustrations.

1. Placing your weight on the balls of your feet, begin to turn your back to the mirror—slowly. Do not lift the feet off the floor. Continuing your turn slowly, with your weight still on the balls of the feet, your back will be to the mirror.

2. With your back to the mirror and in a model's stance, slowly return to face the mirror. Return as before, turning on the balls of your feet.

Let's try it again. Shall we start with our right foot behind us and our left foot pointing to the mirror? All right. When you turn, your left foot will be behind you and your right toe will be pointing straight ahead and should be about 2 inches in front. Until you get complete control, you may find your foot farther away on either your right or left side. Put your weight on the balls of your feet, and put your right foot exactly in the center so that your heel—if you brought it back— would hit your instep.

Now, on the balls of your feet, barely skim your heels off the floor. You don't lift them high. Just barely lift them off the floor so that you can turn your back to the mirror, and you should be in a model's stance.

Notice that you're only turning your body *halfway*—from the

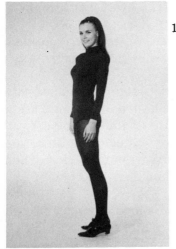

1. Start turning on balls of feet.

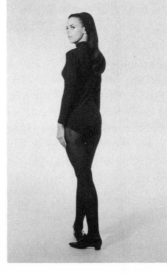

2. Back to mirror. Start turning back, using balls of both feet. Heels barely off floor.

front to the back and from the back to the front. This is your model's
Half Turn.

To turn in *the opposite direction*, you should put your left foot
behind you and point your right toe toward the mirror, then turn on
the balls of your feet. Keep the feet on the floor; they stay there. You
merely turn smoothly, slightly lift your heels off the floor, and your
back will be to the mirror. Now, barely lift the heels off the floor and
return to facing the mirror.

Note: Practice this until you can do it easily. Stay in a model's stance,
and keep your movements smooth. Don't forget: Good posture, tuck
under, control, arms straight down and relaxed.

Model's Walking Pivot or Pivot Four

A model's Walking Pivot combines any number of steps with
a Half Turn. You'll be learning with *four* steps because they are sufficient for practice, and they are a very good number of steps to take
if you are actually modeling onstage.

In your model's stance, step back from your mirror. With your
right foot behind you and your left toe pointing straight ahead, pick
up your front foot. Take one, two, three steps, and on the fourth step,
make it a short one, straight in front of your left toe, and make a Half
Turn to the left. You end up with your right foot behind you.

All right. Let's repeat. Pick up your *left* foot, and one, two, three
steps, and on the fourth step, a short step straight in front, make a
Half Turn, and turn around.

You are completing a circle. Are you aware of that? You are *not*
reversing your turn. You are completing a circle, which is very attractive and flowing, and has a nice feel about it.

Anything that is done in even numbers of steps will cause you
to make and complete a circle. Once you make a turn on the odd step,
it will reverse it. So we call this a Pivot Four. It is a walking pivot; you
can walk any place, and at the end of it when you decide to turn, you
have a Half Turn. But let's practice it as a Pivot Four, so that when
we go into formats you'll understand that when I say, "Pivot Four,"
you'll only take four steps.

Now, let's try the left foot. With your left foot behind you and
your right foot pointing straight ahead (in a model's stance) pick up
your right foot first, then left, right, left. With the left foot directly
in front with that last step (just the length of your shoe because it's
close) you will do a Half Turn and turn around. You will end up with

your left foot behind you and your right foot pointing straight ahead. The right foot should not be way ahead of you. It should only be about 2 inches away. That is why, when you know you're going to make a Half Turn—in any walking pivot—you make your last step a short one so that your feet aren't spread too far apart.

Let's try it again. Left foot behind you, right foot in front and pointing straight ahead — go. One . . . two . . . three . . . short step and turn. The fourth step was the short step.

This is your walking pivot, and we call it a Pivot Four with four steps. Besides being correct when you're modeling onstage, it has the right number of steps to do in the center of a ramp or runway without going too far.

Note: Practice your Pivot Four until you're perfect at it. We'll be using it when we go into the chapter on stage modeling, so have it down pat before you get to it. Start with your right foot first; then practice using your left foot first. Practice until you can glide through the motions with an even, flowing grace.

Model's Pivot and Switching Feet

MODEL'S PIVOT

A Model's Pivot is a turn used in a very small area. When walking up to a person, you would be apt to use this turn. It is used when modeling in tearooms, wholesale showrooms, retail salons, and small areas. It is used in a very small place because you are only taking one small step. It is perfect for television, where space is always at a premium. You can always get out of a tight spot by doing a Model's Pivot.

1. Starting in a model's stance, you will have your weight on your back foot. Always remember: weight on the balls of your feet, never

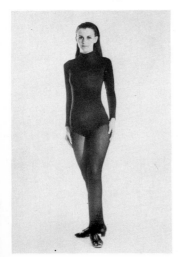

1. Stand in model's stance right foot up-stage, left foot pointing straight ahead. Pick up your left foot in a short step.

heavy on your heels. Your weight is on your back foot, making your front foot look nice and easy, and the muscles relaxed. You would never switch your weight. Your downstage foot will be picked up first in a very short step—just about an inch. Just pick it up and take a short little step in place.

2. Now bring your back foot in front. Notice, your foot is in front of the other and only about an inch away from it. You should feel almost as if you were going to step on your own toes, so that when you turn, you're in a closed-in Model's Pivot. You should not get into the habit of taking too large a step in a Model's Pivot, having your foot possibly 12 inches away from the other foot and being forced to drag it back. The step should be right in place unless you purposely want to make a stride to suit the costume you're wearing.

3. On the balls of both feet, do a Half Turn. You should be in a model's stance, with your back to the audience.

4. Pick up your front foot, then your back foot; repeat. Turn on the balls of both feet, and you'll end up as in Picture 1, with your right foot behind and your left pointing straight to the audience.

Note: This is your model's turn, using the right foot as the upstage

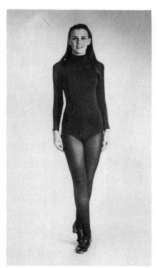 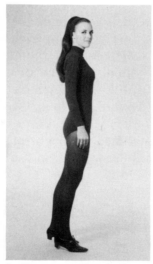 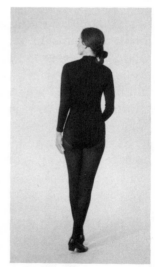

2. Take a short step forward with your right foot. Toe straight ahead.

3. Turn on the balls of both feet to your left, until your back is to audience.

4. Pick up your left foot and then take short step with right foot. Do another Half Turn and you will be around in a model's stance as you began in Picture 1.

foot and the left as the downstage foot. As a time step is to a dancer, so is a Model's Pivot to a 'model. She must know how to do it beautifully, or she will be unable to do any of her other turns well.

Practice putting your left foot behind you and your right foot in front. Always reverse, so that you learn to use both feet. Put your weight on the balls of the feet so that you turn smoothly.

SWITCHING FEET

STEPPING FORWARD ONE STEP. In a model's stance, with your right foot behind you and left foot pointing straight ahead, make a small half-circle with your right foot, pointing it in front of your left foot. Switch your weight to the front foot and turn the back foot in a 45-degree angle so that you will be in a model's stance.

STEPPING BACKWARD ONE STEP. In a model's stance, with the left foot behind you, straighten the back foot by turning to the left on the ball of the foot. Take your front foot and, in a small half-circle, bring it behind your left foot in a 45-degree angle to return to a model's stance.

Note: Be sure that you barely skim the floor with your feet. Use this procedure if you have to take a step forward or backward onstage, or to change position in walking after completing a Model's Pivot. You may need this in tearoom, salon, or television modeling.

Three-Quarter French Turn

The Three-Quarter French Turn is now replacing the Model's Pivot in stage modeling. It has more continuity, and is lovely to look at. Also, you never need worry about the foot being in the wrong walking position.

Let's look at the pictures carefully, and follow them closely.

Starting position: model's stance, left foot behind you. You are at Stage Right. Your right foot is in front of you, and you are ready to turn left on the ball of your back foot, a one-quarter turn so that you are now facing Stage Left. Starting with the left foot, proceed to Stage Left and continue walking.

Because a model keeps her weight on the balls of her feet, it should not look like an awkward cross-over when she picks up her front foot. I'd also like to emphasize the importance of that front foot. In modeling, the important thing is for a girl to look beautiful. And when you step in front of an audience and attempt to take a step with your back foot—as in a model's stance—your legs would be spread apart and not look well at all. Once the body is turned sideways to the audience, it doesn't matter if it's your front or your back foot.

Going back . . . you now are at Stage Right, with your left foot behind you and your right foot in front. As you turn, your whole body turns on the balls of your feet and you start to walk toward the left side of the stage. Now, as you reach Stage Left, you're going to do a Three-Quarter French Turn.

1. You are now at Stage Left. With your right (downstage) foot—your knees and thighs are always close together—you reach around in one continuous motion so that your right foot actually makes a half-circle.
2. Your back will now be to your audience.
3. By placing your weight on the balls of both feet, keep turning on the balls of your feet to show the side of the costume.
4. You will end up in the model's stance. Facing your audience, you are now at Stage Left, with your right foot behind you and your left foot pointed straight ahead.

Note: Practice walking over from Stage Left to Stage Right. It needn't be a long area—about a half-dozen steps will do—just enough to give

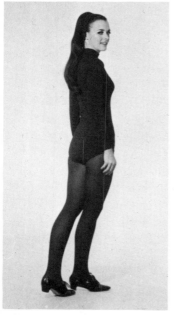

1. Reach around in a half circle with your downstage foot.

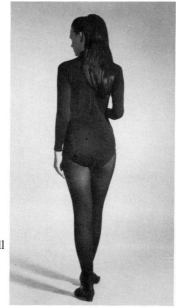

2. Turn on balls of feet. Your back will be to audience. Continue turning . . .

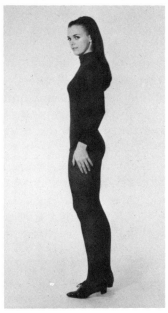

3. . . . As you continue turning, you will now show the side of costume. End up facing the audience in a model's stance as in Picture 4.

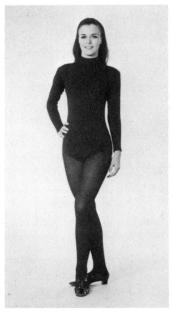

4. You will always end up in a model's stance when completing this turn.

you the feel of walking from one side of the stage to the other.

Turn on the ball of your left foot, and simultaneously get started with your walk by picking up your right (downstage) foot and walk over to Stage Right. As you reach Stage Right, your downstage foot will be your left foot, the one closer to the audience.

Reach around in a half-circle and—in the process of reaching around to do your Three-Quarter French Turn—your shoulders move, the ball of your right (upstage) foot starts to move, and your head moves around. The whole body should be in a flowing motion throughout.

Why do we call it a Three-Quarter French Turn? Because your audience is seeing first the side of your costume, then the back, the other side, and then the front—but your body has only gone *three quarters* of the way. You would have to go another quarter to consider it a full turn.

Practice using hand positions to coordinate smoothly with your Three-Quarter French Turn.

European Turns

EUROPEAN TURN

A European Turn is used effectively in the center of a stage or a runway, or just prior to exits, to do a full-circle turn and continue walking in the same direction. Its purpose is to break the monotony of the walk while continuing in the same direction. It also provides a full view of the costume being modeled.

Practice carefully for a smooth, continuous motion. Never spin or do the turn too rapidly. The object is to display the back, front, and sides of the costume.

Let's pretend you are walking from Stage Left to Stage Right, and you are now in the middle of the stage. Follow the pictures carefully.

1. Reach out with the right foot, pointing the toe out to cut off some of the turn.
2. Cross over with the left foot, keeping as close in as possible, knees touching. The front of the right knee will be touching the back of the left knee. Keep your toe pointing straight ahead.

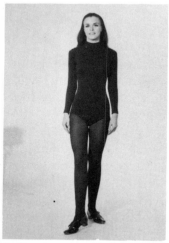

1. Reach out with right foot, point toe out to help cut off some of the turn.

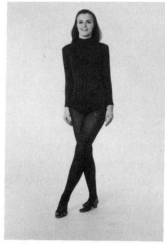

2. Cross over with left leg. Keep legs close, and start turning on the balls of both feet.

3. Turn on the balls of both feet to your right.

4. You will have completed a full-circle turn. Your legs will be crossed rather tightly, and your right foot will be in front. (*Note:* If you find yourself facing the opposite direction, you simply haven't turned far enough. Try again.)

5. Reach out with your right foot and continue walking to the other side of the stage. Actually, at the point where you have completed the full-circle turn you pick up the front foot to avoid a noticeable locking of legs. This is important to practice. When you reach Stage Right, do a Three-Quarter French Turn. Don't forget the left foot is your downstage foot, if you wish to turn and face the audience. Always turn on the balls of both feet. Turn your head slowly to keep contact with your audience. Always maintain a continuous flow of motion.

Note: If you find you have reached an awkward point when your turn is approximately three-quarters completed, pick up your right foot (which will be in front) and continue walking in the direction you are going.

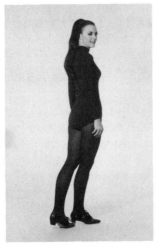

3. Showing how you are turning on balls of feet.

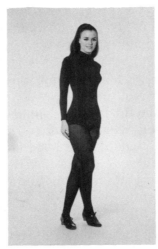

4. You have completed a 360-degree turn and your right leg is in a tight scissor crossover.

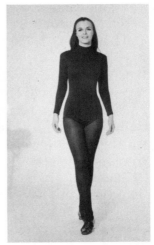

5. Pick up your front foot (it is right in picture) and continue walking to next turning point.

EUROPEAN TURN AND A HALF

A European Turn and a Half is done at the end of a runway. It can also be used as a beautiful exit. The principle behind it is that you can do a complete turn ending up the way you were, and still make another half-turn back the way you were walking, all in one continuous motion. In other words, when you get down to the end of the runway, if you did a *complete* turn, you would still be facing the end of the runway. But with a turn and a half, you would be able to walk back in the opposite direction, so that you can go back on the runway without actually stopping. With flowing chiffons and formals, this can be very effective.

The European Turn and a Half can be very useful in providing an extra turn for the commentary. Let's imagine you are at your exit and realize you should remain onstage longer. Walk over to the center of the stage and do this turn, and then proceed to exit. This is just one example.

If you have to walk offstage into an audience and come back on Stage Right and exit at Stage Right, you will find this turn effective.

Now, the trick to this is that as you come to the end of a runway, point your toe at a 45-degree angle to cut off a good quarter, so that when you reach over with your foot—turning on the balls of your feet—you make a complete turn and a half. Your legs actually get twisted, you pick up your front foot, and continue walking back the way you came.

Using your mirror, try this. Pretend you are at the end of a runway and point your right toe out 45 degrees.

1. Cross over with your left foot, keeping knees and thighs close. Start turning on balls of both feet until . . .
2. You will have turned a full turn and almost another half turn. Your right foot will be crossed over your left. It may be necessary to give a little more turn on the ball of your left foot to propel you around to complete the last half turn.
3. Immediately pick up your right foot and continue walking in the direction you came from.

You will find with practice that you can learn to use your shoulders and the balls of your feet well enough so that you will be making one and a half turns effortlessly. Remember, the object is to have no hesitation.

The European Turn and a Half will be a tricky one to learn. You must keep your knees flexed and have full control of your upper thighs and derriere. This turn is used by all top fashion models, and it gives

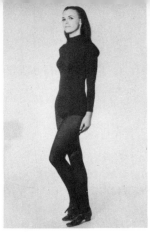 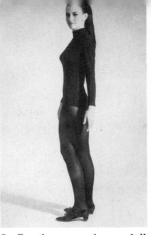 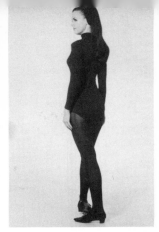

1. After stepping out with your right foot, cross over with your left foot and start turning on the balls of your feet.

2. Continue turning a full turn and a half. As your legs begin to twist and scissor lock you may have to give your left foot a bit more push to get you around.

3. Immediately pick up your right foot and continue walking in the direction you came from. This turn may be done with either foot. Try both, and stick to the one that seems easier for you.

a stunning effect. Don't forget that you have a head and let it follow through with ease. Avoid being stiff and jerky with any part of the body.

Note: Practice in front of your mirror. Keep on stopping, crossing, and turning until you can accomplish the turns in one continuous, fluid motion, and continue walking without stopping. When you can do this easily, without any effort, you'll make your European Turn and a Half with confidence and grace.

DOUBLE EUROPEAN TURN or DOUBLE MILITARY TURN

Step out with your right foot in the same manner as you would start a European Turn. Using the left foot for propulsion, whirl to the right on the ball of the right foot. As you make the 360-degree turn, hold out your left leg with the knee straight and the toe deliberately up. Keep the body straight, as well as the neck and head, keeping arms straight down the side and slightly away from the body to show the silhouette of the costume. Keep the elbows straight and hands up, with palms to the floor.

Complete the turn and take a step with the left foot, and with the next right step do another Military Turn. The two whirl-type turns will make your pleats flare out with great zip. Remember: Only *one* step between. Continue walking and modeling. I feel it is always best to do any unusual turn only once, as too much repetition spoils the effect.

Note: If you feel your costume warrants one more swirl, don't hesitate to do a Double European Turn smoothly and slowly.

Sports Turns

SPORTS STANCE or WIDE-LEG HALF TURN

When a model is showing slacks or any type of pants, like Capris—
bell-bottoms or whatever they are called in any particular year—she
may go into a sports stance when she steps onstage. This will graphically illustrate the way the pants fit the leg.

1. Step out onstage and go into a sports stance. This will show the
tapering, the slimness of the pants, the way they fit, or the way they
bell out, as the case may be. It will give the general outline. If you care
to make a turn and show the back, you will put the weight on the ball
of your downstage foot and merely turn around.
2. You will be in a stance with your back to the audience, as you see
here. I prefer a little bit of an angle to the audience rather than
straight on, but both can be effective. Use your own judgment as to
which you want to use in a given situation.

PIVOT FOUR—SPORTS TURN

In modeling slacks on a stage or on a runway, you can do a Pivot
Four, but with a slight variation. See how it is done in the photographs.

3. As you are centered onstage, do a Pivot Four, but instead of just
turning smoothly and continuing to walk, immediately bend your
knee and lift your heel off the floor. It's the same as a regular Pivot
Four. The only difference lies in the bend of the knee and the lift of
the heel. You could use a picture effect with your hands like our model.
4. As you can see in this picture, when you turn and walk back and
finish your Pivot Four, you will be showing the inside of the leg on the

| 1. Spread the legs. Keep the heels slightly to center. | 2. Turning on the ball of one foot, turn and show the back of pants. | 3. Do a Half Turn and lift front heel off floor. Note hand position. |

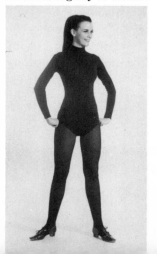
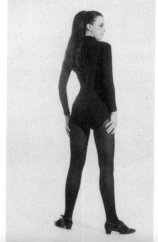
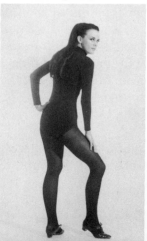

second turn. By the time you've taken four steps, you've shown the outside and the inside of the leg. This is excellent in the center of a stage, walking from Stage Left to Stage Right, or in the center of a runway. Remember: Keep moving even when you are modeling slacks.

THREE-QUARTER FRENCH TURN—END OF RUNWAY

This is a sports turn that utilizes the Three-Quarter French Turn at the end of a runway. It is effective when modeling a sportswear fashion that has a wide skirt. Also use it with any pants or pajamas. This is how you do it.

5. As you reach the end of the runway, with your left foot step to the right corner of the runway. Bring your right foot around in a wide half-circle (turning on the balls of both feet) as you do in a Three-Quarter French Turn. You will have the left foot in front of you, thus giving you a wide spread of the legs. Upon completing the turn, bend the knee and lift the heel of the front foot.

6. With a continuous movement, bring the front leg in a smooth swing forward to start walking back up the runway. This whole process should be smooth and continuous to look right.

Review: There are three versions of the proper handling of pants and slacks. Be sure you learn them all.

1. A stance and then turning around—to show back and front—with the legs spread apart.

2. Doing a Pivot Four, and using your sports turn effect with it.

4. Walk four steps and do a Half Turn again, lifting heel of front foot. Continue walking.	5. Swing around with weight on left foot. Make a deliberate wide step and lift heel to show pants.	6. Immediately swing the leg smoothly in front to continue walking up runway.

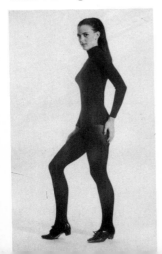 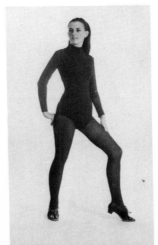 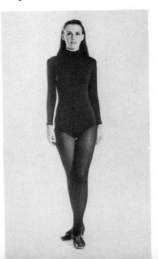

3. Three-Quarter French Sports Turn at end of a runway.

I'd like to remind you that when you are modeling culottes or pants with a full cut, you may have to use your hands to show the line of the pants leg. Don't be afraid to do anything that will effectively show the shape of the leg — pants leg, not yours! — as that is the whole purpose in modeling it.

HAND POSITIONS AND GRACE

Exercises

Using your hands gracefully is a very important part of modeling. You may be beautiful in every other respect, but if your hands are tense and you handle them poorly, you will spoil the complete look you are trying to achieve.

A model will use her hand positions in the process of doing any kind of a turn, to accent the line of the garment. Perhaps she won't use a hand position at all. Her hands will just be down at the sides, and relaxed or lifted away from the body to show the outline or silhouette of the garment, but if she does use her hands on turns, the audience should be unaware of them. You must avoid the monotonous look of hands merely hanging at the sides throughout the showing of a fashion.

Here are some exercises to help you achieve this. Follow the pictures, and don't forget to use your mirror.

1. Squeeze fingers into a tight ball.
2. Stretch fingers open wide.
3. Shake hands vigorously to loosen muscles.
4. This is an exercise, but at the same time it shows you how much

1. Squeeze fingers into a tight ball.   2. Stretch fingers open wide.   3. Shake hands vigorously to loosen muscles.

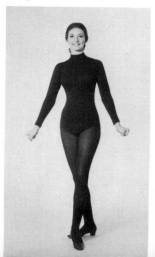 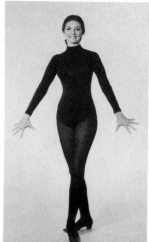 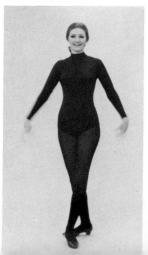

prettier hands look when the sides are to the camera or audience, rather than the back of the hands. Start with your hands up at chest level with fingers curved and graceful, the two center fingers slightly lower. You must lead with the wrist, keeping your hands long, soft, and relaxed.

5. Open your arms, and make a big, wide circle. As you reach up to the ceiling, your palms will be up, facing the ceiling.

6. When your arms are down to shoulder height, turn palms down.

7. Bring your arms down so that the elbows will give a gentle curve. Then come down into what is almost a ballet look, with hands barely touching in front of you. Now gently bring them back up to the chest area, as you see in Picture 4.

See how much prettier your hand looks when you don't boldly show the palm or the back of it. A three-quarter to a side angle is always much more graceful with the hands, but this exercise is just sweeping them up and coming down, and up and out and down.

Another trick I like is to be aware that the wrist should have about a 45-degree angle to the straight of the arm. If you keep it straight, it isn't as pretty. A little hint of gentleness will make it look much lovelier. Here's an exercise that will help.

Place your hand in a ballet position, as if you were going to reach for a marble or a grape. Reach with your thumb and your two center fingers and pick up the grape. Notice how much more gracefully your hand goes into this line. Your little finger and your index finger will be slightly up. To pick up any light object, learn to use your two center fingers and your thumb, and reach as if you're going to pick up an object with your wrist.

You reach with the wrist, and then use the fingers. You don't plow in with the fingers first. Always do hand motions with the wrist. Your

4. Palms down, with arm and hands at shoulder level.	5. Pushing with the wrists, lift arms and hands high above head. Palms up.	6. As you reach shoulder level, turn palms down. Lead with wrists, keep hands soft.
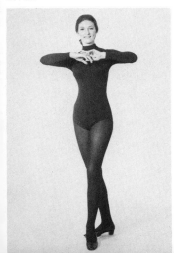	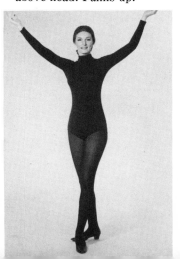	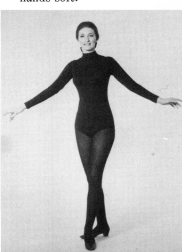

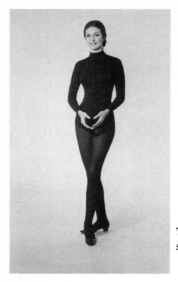

7. Bring relaxed fingers together and start over again as in Picture 4.

hand line will be so much softer if you are aware that the *wrist does the leading.* Always reach up as if the wrist is doing it. Unless you have extremely beautiful hands, avoid showing the complete back of your hands to camera or audience.

Raise your hands high above your head. Rub back of hands toward the elbows. This will smooth protruding veins for a few seconds for camera or stage.

Note: While you are modeling, be aware that you are concentrating on these areas:

1. Lead any hand motion from the wrist, not the fingers.
2. Keep hands relaxed, graceful, and long.
3. Never have all four fingers together or tense.
4. Learn to keep the two center fingers slightly lower on a side view or front view.
5. Pick up any part of your costume with thumb and two center fingers for a light, lovely look.

Using Hand Positions While Modeling

There are basic hand positions that should be adjusted to each garment. They would not be used with everything. As I've already mentioned, 99 percent of the time your hand positions would be done on turns.

Now, stand in front of your mirror and follow the photographs carefully.

1. Asymmetrical hand position. Place your hands as if they were on the seams of your dress, elbows back, side view to the audience. One hand is always slightly higher than the other. Never spread the fingers. The two center fingers are together gently, and the others separated. You actually can't see this from the side view, but it still is important. Hands may turn slightly back or slightly forward. It depends on which looks best. If your hands are a bit bold and strong, you should turn them back toward the derriere. This will give a more slenderizing line, which will be prettier. Hands that are very slender and lovely can turn more forward.

2. One hand on the waist. If this were a garment where your elbows were exposed, be aware that when you use the elbow that corresponds with your upstage foot, you'll get a softer line, fingers forward, thumb back, wrist dropped and relaxed.

3. Place both hands on waist. Now you see what I mean about the sharp elbow! It might be wise to have that effect, but with the other arm down. You can always have a left or a right arm up on the waist and the other one down. The hand is placed on a line of the garment. If you want to emphasize the waist or a belt line, this would be fine. But if the gar-

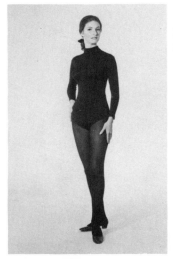

1. Asymmetrical hand position. Hands down side seam of dress. One hand higher.

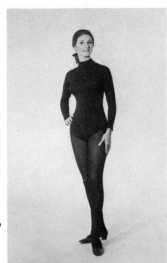

2. One hand at line of costume. Keep wrist and fingers relaxed.

ment is a hipbone-length jacket or has a belt elsewhere than at the waist, the hand should be at the line of the garment.

Sometimes there is controversy about using hands directly across from each other, but there are times when it can be very effective, especially when we have a very small-waisted model and she wants to emphasize the small waistline by putting both hands on her waist. This can be done occasionally for effect, but not often.

4. This is the classic position with hands on derriere. You get a very gentle roundness to the elbows, so that you achieve a complete silhouette, and no hands are in the way to destroy the look.

5. This is your sports stance. You will see it—and its variations—in the fashion magazines. When a model puts her knuckles into a sports stance, notice that the little finger is toward the audience or camera, to show the side view of the hands. The wrist is dropped, not stiff, but you'll observe that it has a 45-degree angle to the arm. With the sports hand position, if the whole back of the hand is to the camera, you get a "clump" look, which is not attractive at all.

Look in the mirror and check for yourself what a difference it makes. You must always be conscious of pretty lines with arms and hands. Anything that is done with two hands can be done with one, as we see in . . .

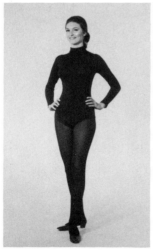
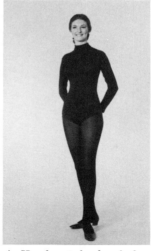
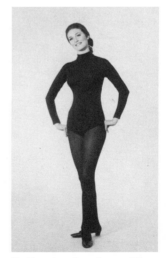

3. Both hands on waist, or line of garment.

4. Hands at back of derriere. Important to show a waistline.

5. Sports hand position. Wrists dropped and side of hand showing.

6. . . . One hand down and the other in a sports hand position. This would be effective in turning a sport jacket back and emphasizing a slim skirt on a turn.

7. This is how a girl should look when she turns and is actually walking away. She would be on a runway, looking left and right, or turning onstage with her back to the audience, keeping her arm close to her body. Bringing one arm gently in front like this in a curve is most effective. She might even lift it—as in Picture 7—when she walks away from the audience, showing, for instance, the back of a jacket, arms down, and how it looks when the arm is bent.

You are selling clothes and showing their effectiveness. You have to sit, you have to move, in clothes. When you see that they look well in motion, you can sell them.

8. There will be an occasion when you may want to lift an arm on a turn, or, possibly, when walking. Lift the arm below the bust line. At this height you will not show a bulge of muscles. A girl who is very thin may lift an arm higher. However, the hand looks best either below or above the bust line. When you are bringing your hand up, you will find that the hand will look prettier if the palm is down. There should be a lightness in the hand, and the wrist should be at an approximate 45-degree angle to the hand. Fingers should be toward the audience or camera, with a front view.

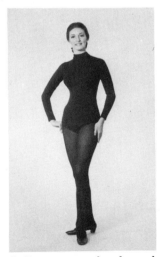 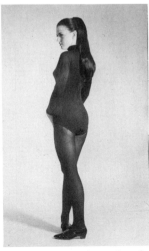 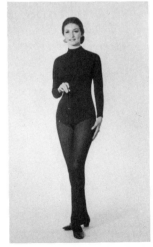

6. Drop one hand and use the other for a sports look.	7. Bringing the hands gently in front of upper thighs will soften elbows on some turns.	8. Raise one hand gracefully under bustline. Fingers forward and arm close and easy to body.

9. Be aware that you use your hands gracefully on jackets. You should come in and hold the edge of the jacket with the two center fingers and a thumb, let your elbows go back and your hands fall back in a graceful line. This depicts a graceful look with the hands, especially when wearing a delicate fabric.

10. If you are modeling a tailored jacket of a sturdier fabric, do not clutch the jacket with thumb and index finger. Use your center fingers to hold the edge at the hipline joint.

11. Bring your arm up very gently on the jacket, and get this nice three-quarter view of the hand. Bring the arm back, place your hand properly at the waist, let the wrist relax and the fingers look long and slim. You must learn to use your hands with a natural elegance.

12. To emphasize a smaller waist, use the thumbs to bring it in. This isn't used as often as Picture 13. When fingers are forward and wrists are dropped, you get a prettier line; also, a look of sharp elbows is less evident. Yet there is a need for both these hand positions. You will find more use for 13 than for 12, because it is more flattering to the arm and wrist and is less cramped.

14. With a jacket—removing it or just showing the shoulder line of the blouse underneath—your hands must be graceful. Do not grab, or push, or look forceful. It's just a nice easy use of center fingers and thumbs, and showing the shoulder line. Use the same procedure in lifting the jacket back up on the shoulders, always being careful to use your hands in a graceful manner.

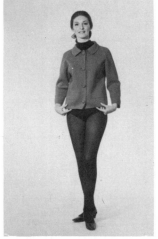 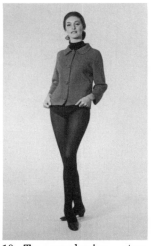 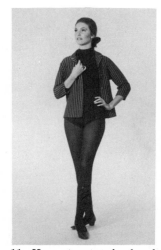

9. Hold edge of jacket with two center fingers and thumb. Do this at the hip-bone area.

10. To emphasize sturdier fabrics use the hands with more strength.

11. How to touch lapel gracefully and open one side of coat or jacket.

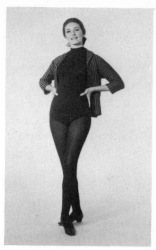
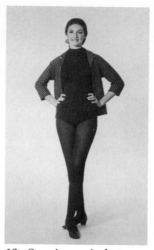
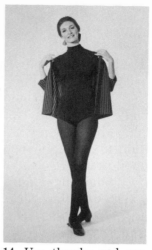

12. Thumbs forward and fingers down side seam of costume.

13. Opening jacket or coat with fingers forward, wrists dropped. Jacket off bustline.

14. Use thumbs and center fingers of each hand to gracefully lift jacket off shoulder to show line of sleeve.

Note: With your mirror as an ally, practice using your hand positions until you can do them with ease. It is very easy to have an ugly hand position. There are all types of clothes, and the hand position must be adjusted to each costume and its line. You must realize that the main object is to be able to use your hands gracefully, and thus handle any costume with ease and confidence.

EXPRESSION AND PERSONALITY

To Smile—or Not to Smile

That is the question! Smiling is to warm the audience to what you wear, to show them that *you* love it. However, everything doesn't sell because you smile. If you're showing fun clothes, you'd be apt to smile. If the costume is sophisticated, there can be a slight smile on your face, but not a toothy grin. If you are allowed to perform as you like, make your own decision according to what you're wearing. Does it require a smile? Will it sell better if you smile?

Actually, it depends on your employer. With wholesale modeling, of course, a smile isn't necessary. The buyers are business people. They are buying clothes, and their eyes are only on the clothes as you whisk in and out. In some showrooms, informality is the order of the day.

In a plush salon where the showing would be exclusive, a model rarely smiles. Her business is strictly to *show the garment*, and either the fashion coordinator or the director of the salon will be selling the clients. At that time, the model is a true mannequin.

In a spring fashion show, one of our models smiled. She was the only one who did. Upon being questioned, she said she had just decided she felt like smiling in what she was wearing. Since she was in a position to do what she liked, it was quite acceptable. She smiled. Nine models didn't—and one did.

Some designers—not all—feel that a smile detracts from the garment. It has become rather common for models not to smile in most fashion shows because they want all the attention on the garment, and an attractive smile might detract. On the other hand, in informal modeling, a smile may relax the audience and show the model's inner feelings toward the garment, and this will sell it better. So, it's rather a case of mixed emotions, and letting your instinct be your guide. The one girl who smiled in the fashion show I mentioned wanted to be different—and she *was* different. But this doesn't mean that every girl is going to go out and decide, "I'm going to smile."

It still comes back to what you're wearing. You must learn to understand the feeling of clothes and the emotion of clothes. You must know that a self-assured model with a carefree look and an air of complete ease and confidence often sells the fashion better than the one who is smiling.

You'll really have to think about the "feel" of a costume before you decide on your expression. If it's gay—and the designer allows it—then smile. If it's very high style, look dignified. Naturally, there are all kinds of costumes and expressions in between.

Note: Practice your expressions before your mirror. Every model practices expressions in front of a mirror privately. Learn to know your best expressions, but change them to suit the mood of the costume. Have a collection of the latest fashion magazines on hand, and compare. Match your expressions to the ones the models are wearing when you model similar clothes.

ENTRANCES AND EXITS

Stage Entrances

Walk to the point where you are told to make your stage entrance. At times there will be archways; at other times there will be a platform to step up on. Stages vary. If it is a conventional stage, walk to the center of it. A model's stance, with your upstage foot, is appropriate, then place your hands in whatever position is necessary for the garment.

A more beautiful entrance—and one you would probably use more often—is a Three-Quarter French Turn entrance. This is walking to the center of the stage, or wherever directed, and reaching around with your downstage foot. Continue walking downstage. You can see how this is done in the next chapter.

Stage Exits

HALF-TURN EXIT

Now it's time to talk about exits. How do you get off the stage gracefully?

Let's pretend—before we even go into a format—that you are walking upstage from the footlights on Stage Right, and that you're going to go off on Stage Right.

As you reach the back of the stage, simply do a Half Turn to your exit. You will be facing the audience in a model's stance. Then, turning on the balls of your feet, you will walk offstage. That is your Half Turn exit. You may also take your downstage foot and pose it out in a three-o'clock position or some other fashion pose before turning and walking offstage.

THREE-QUARTER FRENCH-TURN EXIT

If you want a more flowing exit, you will find that a Three-Quarter French Turn exit is more graceful. You are at Stage Right. Walk from the footlights to the back of the stage and reach with the left foot pointing toward the center of the audience. This will place your body sideways when walking offstage.

Always practice your exits on both Stage Right and Stage Left.

EUROPEAN-TURN EXIT

You may use a European Turn for exits. If you are at Stage Right downstage and you're to exit at Stage Left, you can actually make an angle upstage, walking back to the center, and do a European Turn, especially if it is a large stage. When you are about three-quarters of the way, or close, to the exit, do another European Turn and continue walking off. Your side will be to the audience, not your back.

Never turn your back to the audience and walk off. Always give the impression that you are with it all the way, by turning at least one time to the audience before turning sideways or turning your back.

Note: Practice your exits at Stage Left and Stage Right, using a Half Turn to your audience, a Three-Quarter French Turn, reaching with the foot so that you'll go to the center of the stage and then end up walking offstage sideways. If you are on the opposite side of the stage, walk directly toward your exit doing a European Turn—one or two, if necessary—and continue walking.

STAIRS AND SITTING

How to Go Up and Down Stairs

Occasionally you'll be involved in a fashion show that uses stairs. It may only include the two or three steps you'll need to get up onto your runway, or it may be a whole flight of steps that forms an integral part of an elaborate production. Going up and down these steps gracefully, and with assurance, is important.

The correct approach is essential. You measure with your eyes to get an idea of the distance. You don't bend your head, but just glance down.

1. Place your entire foot on the step, not just the front part with the heel lapping over. Your thigh and knee joints are what really do the smooth walking up the stairs. You will go up easily. Whether you start with your upstage or downstage foot depends on the gown you'll be showing. Which will look better? Look in a mirror and see which one would.

Pose at the top of the stairs, unless you're going to continue moving. In that case, do a Three-Quarter French Turn and glide on down the stairs.

2. It's the descent that is particularly noticed when a model does it poorly. Your knees should touch gently as you start down the stairs. Your knees are flexed and bent. You reach with your toe, and your heel eases down. Your eyes stay up and you look straight ahead.

3. You'll feel this with your foot, and there is literally quite a bend to the knee. It's a tucking under and a bend. Practice this until you feel a tremendous gliding. If you were walking this way on a level surface in a room, you would practically be walking in a semi-crouch.

Note: Practice this. It's actually very amusing when we practice this in class. We practice bending our knees and walking around the room to get the feeling of how you bend your knees and keep them bent as you glide down the stairs.

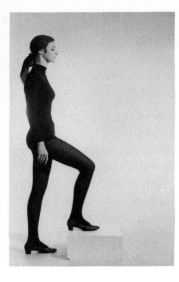

1. Place complete foot on step to avoid an accident. Lower eyes, but not head.

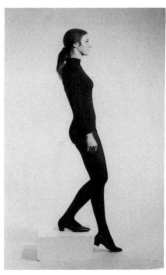

2. Reach and feel step with toe of shoe. Ease the heel down, keeping knees bent for a gliding motion. Note head is up, and knees will touch as you glide down.

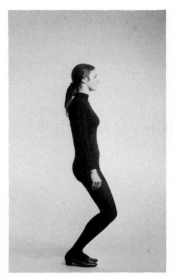

3. Tuck under firmly, bend the knees, and walk around the room for practice. You should feel this way while descending stairs.

How to Sit

A model should know how to sit properly. You may be required to be seated on a stage at times, and the lovely effect should not be spoiled by being clumsy. There's a right way to do this.

Gracefully and easily lower your body, with your knees together and one foot ahead of the other. Try to create a soft S-line. It's a more graceful look. The whole approach is to sit with ease, and immediately go into a position of natural grace. You may be asked to sit up on a high stool, or any high object. Your knees must be together; one foot is advanced or crossed at the ankle; both feet are fairly close to each other, and your hands are positioned softly and elegantly.

You never use your hands to pull yourself out of a chair. Hands should be placed on front of upper thighs to give your body assistance in rising. You allow your body to do this. Rise fluidly and in one easy motion.

Note: If you practice your sitting and standing whenever you have to do so ordinarily, you'll soon learn to do it properly for the stage. Also check sitting position for "Bathing Suits" in Chapter 8 on "Fashion Photography."

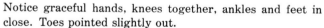

Notice graceful hands, knees together, ankles and feet in close. Toes pointed slightly out.

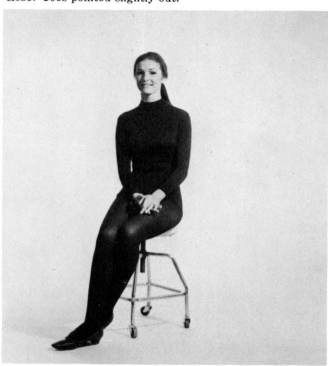

4.

STAGE MODELING MADE EASY

As a professional model, you will rarely have a rehearsal before a fashion show. This would cost the producers extra money and you are expected to know how to work on a stage under ordinary circumstances. If, however, the producers are planning something unusual and want to be certain it comes off smoothly, you can expect a rehearsal. Rehearsal time will vary from an hour or more, depending on production needs.

You have already learned your various model turns. We will now abbreviate the names of the turns to their initials. Do you recognize them?

½ T. .... One-Half Turn
¾ F. T. .... Three-Quarter French Turn
E. T. .... European Turn
E. T. & ½ ..... European Turn and a Half
P. 4 .... Pivot Four (walking four steps and Half Turn)
M.P. .... Model's Pivot (although not used in stage formats)

When you arrive backstage for a fashion show, and you have your clothes and accessories lined up, you will then want to take a quick look at the stage. Size up the width and length carefully and work out a visual format. If it is at all possible to practice on the stage, do so. You may have to ask permission from the fashion coordinator, with whom you have first checked in. Every stage has a different feel and you will be more comfortable if you know it. This is not always possible, however.

On the following page you will find two diagrams. They represent your first stage format. The filled-in one is an example only. You will learn by working in the *blank* stage.

Note: The audience, Stage Left, and Stage Right always remain the same. When you are standing on a stage and are facing the audience, Stage Right is to *your* right, and Stage Left is to *your* left. When you turn your back to the audience, this is reversed.

FORMAT A

Format A may be used for any type of costume or coat. Excellent for slacks and sport clothes.

ASSIGNMENT

Copy the filled-in stage format on the diagram of the blank stage. Take your pencil and do not lift it off the paper. Start at your entrance on Stage Left. Follow the numbers and let the pencil do the turns. This will give you the feeling of smoothness that we want you to achieve when you're modeling onstage.

Now it is your turn to do it personally. Establish your audience in your practice room. Walk over to Stage Left and practice your Format A. Walk through it slowly at first, and then begin modeling with all the techniques you've learned from the previous chapters.

Explanation of Format A

Have someone read this aloud while you model Format A, or read it yourself while you are walking through the format.

Format A

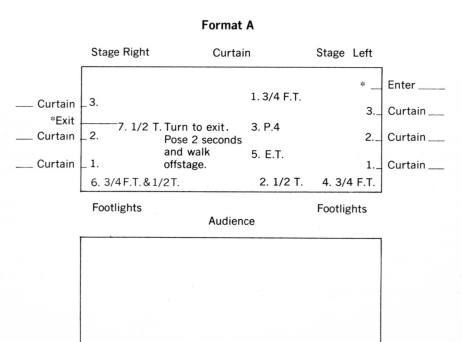

We shall assume that the stage has three curtains and you are standing in the wings off Stage Left behind curtain No. 3.

1. Walk to Center Stage and reach with your downstage foot (the one nearer your audience, remember?) and do a Three-Quarter French Turn. You should be facing your audience.

2. Walk straight down to the footlights and do a Half Turn, which faces you toward the back of the stage.

3. Keep walking backstage four steps to complete a Pivot Four.

4. Walk down to the corner at Stage Left, reach around with your downstage foot and do a Three-Quarter French Turn. You should be facing your audience in a model's stance, with your left foot downstage. Your downstage foot always takes the first step.

5. Start walking over to Stage Right and as you reach Center Stage, do a European Turn and continue on to Stage Right.

6. At Stage Right, reach with your downstage foot and do another Three-Quarter French Turn. You should be facing your audience. Take a short step straight ahead and do a Half Turn.

7. Walk back beyond Curtain No. 2 (Stage Right), take a short step with your right foot, turning toward your exit and back to your audience with a Half Turn. You should be in a model's stance with your left foot downstage. Lift your left foot in a natural walking position, and your right foot will turn slightly as you walk off the stage.

Note: Be sure that you are turning on the balls of your feet to keep everything moving in your pivots and turns.

1. Know all your pivots and turns before you begin.

2. Practice using your hand positions carefully on turns.

3. Practice expression with your eyes and mouth.

4. Don't forget that you do have a head and keep it turned slightly toward the audience.

5. Look beautiful and feel confident.

Do you have the feel of it now? Your living room can be a practice stage for you, and you can invite your friends and/or relatives to be your audience. Start slowly, and walk and do your turns with Format A as though you were onstage. Practice, practice, practice until you don't have to think consciously of the format.

Now we reverse the entrance and the exit. Walk to Stage Right and do your complete Format A, only this time you exit at Stage Left. You must learn to work both sides of your stage.

Let's review the areas you want to perfect:

1. Walk smoothly, quickly, and turn slowly.
2. Keep your arms and hands relaxed when walking.
3. Use your hands to show the line of your costume on your turns.
4. Hold your head beautifully and turn it to look at your audience.
5. Have a pleasant expression on your face, and keep your eyes alert and interested.
6. Exchange the E. T. Center Stage for a P. 4 Sports Turn if modeling slacks.

If you have a record player, buy some instrumental records and practice to music. Or you can turn on the radio and practice to all types of music. You should be able to model to whatever musical beat is current. The usual type of tunes played at fashion shows is cocktail music, but it is no longer unusual to stage a showing of very young clothes to the rhythms of a modern group. For fun clothes, it's fun music!

On the following pages, you will find Format B, Format C, and Format D. Fill in the blank stages and then practice with the pencil before you get up and actually model as if you were onstage. You will very soon find that you have the feel for the various types of staging.

Don't forget: Always reverse your practice as you learn each of the formats printed on these pages. You never know from which side of the stage you will enter or exit until you arrive backstage, so feel comfortable on either side.

FORMAT B

Format B is excellent for formals, chiffons, flowing fabrics that move easily.

ASSIGNMENT

Copy Format B in your blank stage. Again, take your pencil and do not lift it off the paper.

Note: In Format A we showed you a stage with Curtains Nos. 1, 2, and 3. A model will never know between which curtains she is expected to enter or exit until she is directed. Some stages have fewer than three curtains. They are usually different in color, and the director may tell you to enter in front of a pink curtain rather than a number. These curtains are the wings of a stage, and you often will hear this expression.

Explanation of Format B

1. Entering from Stage Left, walk down to Center Stage and do a European Turn.

Format B

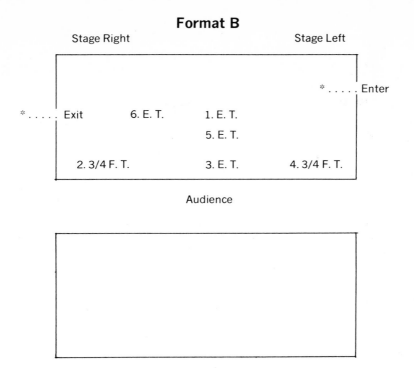

Stage Right   Stage Left

*..... Enter

*..... Exit   6. E. T.   1. E. T.

5. E. T.

2. 3/4 F. T.   3. E. T.   4. 3/4 F. T.

Audience

2. Walk down to Stage Right, reach with your downstage foot and do a Three-Quarter French Turn. You should be facing your audience.

3. Walk straight over to Center Stage and do a European Turn.

4. Continue walking to Stage Left, reach with your downstage foot and do a Three-Quarter French Turn. You should be facing your audience.

5. Walk at an angle back to Center Stage and do a European Turn.

6. Keep walking toward your exit (Stage Right) and do another European Turn before you exit.

Since this book is your instructor, we feel it necessary to repeat reminders. You, too, must remind yourself constantly about major points of modeling.

1. If you are modeling a formal with Format B, you will hold your arms easy and out on your turns—away from the body—to show the silhouette of the gown. Remember to think that you have *no* hands. They must be long, graceful, and completely relaxed. If the skirt is very full, you should ease your arms away from your body so that they won't be hanging into the folds of the skirt on a turn. Should the skirt be cut straight, your hands could hang naturally and straight from

the shoulder. You will use your arms and hands to move the chiffon formals.

2. Remember that you do have an audience, so move your neck slightly to turn and look at that audience. Have you ever seen a fashion model who never moves her head or neck? It appears very tense and most unnatural.

3. Are you taking approximately eight to ten steps within five seconds? Your walk should not be slow. If the stage is very small, you will slow down your pace accordingly.

4. Are you checking your walk to be certain you are not toeing in—or out—too much?

FORMAT C

This format is excellent for coats, formals with evening coats, and for every costume that features back interest.

ASSIGNMENT

Take your pencil and draw Format C in your blank stage. Follow your format closely.

Note: You will notice that each of your exits has been different.

1. When you are on the opposite side of the stage from which you will be exiting, you will find that European Turns in Center Stage

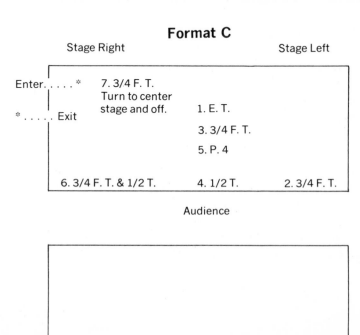

Format C

Audience

and close to the exit will be best. If the stage is short, do one European Turn.

2. If you plan to exit offstage from the same side on which you have done your last turn, you will do a Half Turn or a Three-Quarter French Turn: Half Turn for a last-minute posing; Three-Quarter French Turn for a continuous flowing exit.

Explanation of Format C

1. Entering from Stage Right and walking to Center Stage, do a European Turn slowly and smoothly.

2. Continue to walk to Stage Left and reach with your downstage foot and do a Three-Quarter French Turn. You should be facing your audience.

3. Angle back to Center Stage and reach with your downstage foot to do another Three-Quarter French Turn. You should be facing the audience Center Stage.

4. Walk straight down Center Stage to the footlights and do a Half Turn.

5. Walk straight back Stage Center four steps to complete a Pivot Four.

6. Walk down to Stage Right and reach with your downstage foot and do a Three-Quarter French Turn. Step forward one step to do a Half Turn.

7. Walk upstage to the point where you will want to exit. Reach around with your left foot and do a Three-Quarter French Turn. Notice you are turning to Center Stage and your audience; continue to turn toward your exit and walk off Stage Right.

Note: 1. If you were using this format to remove a jacket, start unbuttoning it as you finish your Three-Quarter French Turn on 2, Stage Left. This should allow you sufficient time to unbutton and have your jacket open to show what is underneath, as you complete your Three-Quarter French Turn at Center Stage, 3. The jacket can be removed as you are walking down Center Stage to 4. If you keep moving, you will have enough time to remove a jacket smoothly, and have it appear effortless. You will need to practice this often to acquire the right timing for various types of jackets and coats.

2. Are you remembering to keep moving? Clothes are more beautiful in motion. The audience has seen enough by the time you have covered the stage.

FORMAT D

This format is excellent for any costume that has back interest.

ASSIGNMENT

Copy Stage Format D in your blank stage. Follow the moves with your pencil.

Note: You will now practice your Three-Quarter French Turns on Stage Left and Stage Right, using your upstage foot. Your back will be to the audience and you continue to walk, completing a Pivot Four.

I would suggest that you do not try to master this format until you have the first three formats under control.

Format D

Stage Right			Stage Left
1. 3/4 F. T.			* . . . . . Enter
	8. E. T.	Exit . . . . . *	
7. P. 4	5. E. T.	4. P. 4	
6. 3/4 F. T. Upstage foot	2. 3/4 F. T.	3. 3/4 F. T. Upstage foot	

Audience

A professional model must learn to use both feet in her turns. You achieve a different position of the body toward the audience when you learn to do your turns with both feet.

Remember to always follow through from one point to the next with grace. Use your stage with ease.

Explanation of Format D

1. Enter from Stage Left. Walk to Center Stage and reach with your downstage foot and do a Three-Quarter French Turn.

2. Walk straight down Stage Center to the footlights and reach around with your left foot to do a Three-Quarter French Turn. You should be facing Stage Left.

3. Walk over to the corner of Stage Left, and this time reach with your upstage foot to do a Three-Quarter French Turn. You will have your back to the audience.

4. Continue to walk straight upstage four steps to complete a Pivot Four.

5. Walk over to Center Stage and do a European Turn.

6. Continue to walk down to Stage Right and again reach with your upstage foot to do a Three-Quarter French Turn. You will have your back to the audience.

7. Walk straight back to Stage Right and finish with a Pivot Four.

8. Walk over to Stage Left gracefully and work your way upstage to the point where you plan to exit. Do a European Turn just past Center Stage. Do not stop, just keep going off Stage Left and exit.

Note: 1. Any costume that has back interest will show effectively with Format D. You are showing the back of the garment on both Stage Right and Stage Left.

2. Now that you have practiced using your upstage foot to do your Three-Quarter French Turns, you can see where they could be exchanged with any other format.

SPECIAL ASSIGNMENT

Take all of your turns and mix them into a stage format of your own. Do at least one variation from what you have learned. Keep in mind that you must make a turn of some type on Stage Left, Stage Right, and Center Stage. You would be cheating your audience if you missed any one of these points.

FASHION SHOW PICTURES

On the following pages are photographs of models at a showing of holiday and resort fashions of 1969, called "Tropicana Holiday Fiesta," at the Tropicana Hotel in Las Vegas. Top designers Malcolm Starr, Adele Simpson, Luis Estevez, Oscar de la Renta, Jean Louis, Royer of Acapulco, and Christian Dior showed their collection. Each designer selected and fitted the models needed for the showing prior to their flying to Las Vegas. The models are from New York, Los Angeles, and San Francisco. New York models are from Frances Gill, Ford, Mannequin, and Paul Wagner model agencies; Los Angeles models, from Mary Webb Davis, Nina Blanchard, and Fran O'Brien model agencies; and San Francisco models, from the Bredner Model Agency.

Please note the positions of the legs, feet, hands, arms, the overall posture, and head positions of each model. Notice the different expressions of the models and their great confidence. Study the ones you like and practice in front of a mirror. Remember, it is an inner feeling as well as an exterior look.

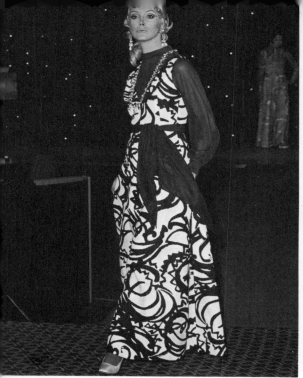

Designer Adele Simpson

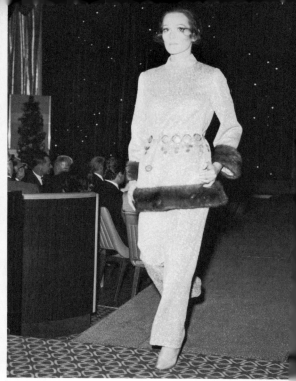

Designer Jean Louis

Designer Jean Louis

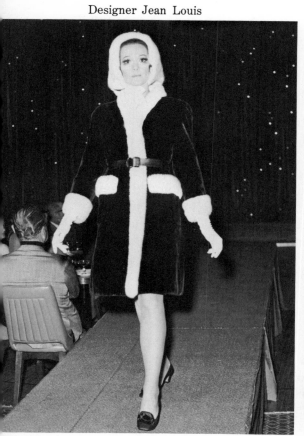

Designer Oscar de la Renta

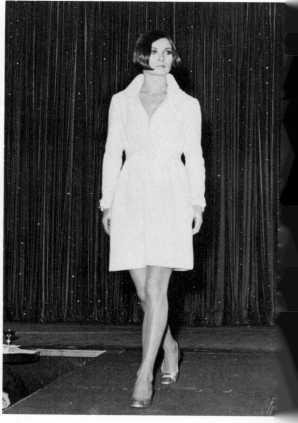

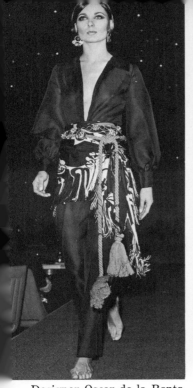
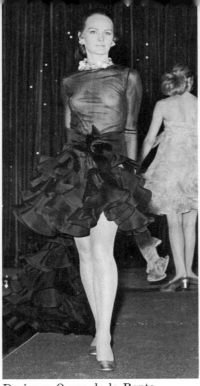
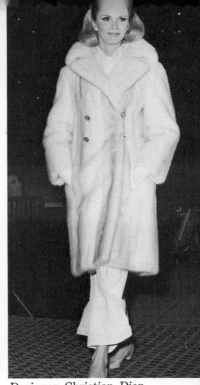

Designer Oscar de la Renta Designer Oscar de la Renta Designer Christian Dior

Designer Christian Dior Designer Christian Dior

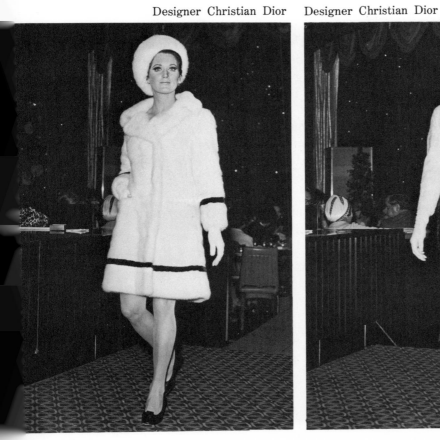
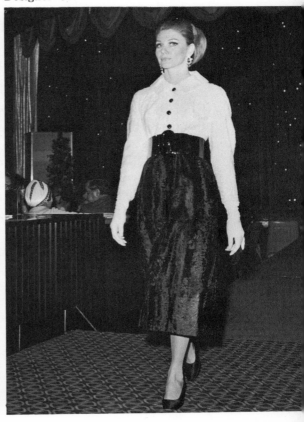

5

RUNWAY MODELING

Runways—or catwalks as they are called in England—are often used for fashion shows. Many rooms do not have a built-in stage, so a runway will be built for the occasion. It is a temporary structure and usually can be dismantled quickly and easily. The material often used for building runways is plyboard, which comes in dimensions of 4 feet by 8 feet. This is why you'll generally see ramps in multiples of 8 feet. They would be 16 feet, 24 feet, 32 feet, and so on.

There are, of course, permanent runways, which can be of any number of shapes. I'm giving you formats for four different types.

There are many different turns that you can mix or match on a runway, but what you'll have to watch especially is where you enter and where you exit.

There usually will be an audience on three or four sides. Therefore, be sure that you're modeling to all sides.

RUNWAY FORMAT A

ASSIGNMENT

As with the stage formats I've given you, copy Runway Format A on the blank runway below it. Take your pencil and do not lift it off the paper. Starting at the stairs, follow the numbers and let the pencil make the turns. Since this runway has steps only at one end, you will make your exit there also.

Now you're ready to actually do this. Establish your audience in your practice room.

Runway Format A

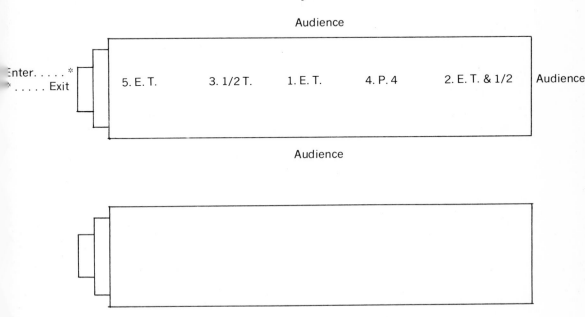

Format A is used when modeling a single garment.

Explanation of Runway Format A

Have someone read this aloud while you model Runway Format A, or read it to yourself while you are walking through the format.

The stairs are at one side only here, so you will enter and exit from the same side. If you are modeling a dress — without a coat or jacket to remove — here is one way you would handle this:

1. Walk to the middle of the ramp and do an easy European Turn.
2. Walk down to the end and slowly do a European Turn and a Half.
3. Walking back just past the center, do a Half Turn.
4. Finish up with four steps for a Pivot Four, which, of course, is another Half Turn with four steps between.
5. Walk down to the stair end of the ramp, do a smooth European Turn and go off.

Note: This is your basic diagram for Runway Format A. Don't forget it all depends on the length of the runway. Runways will vary from 8 to 80 feet in length, and you have to adjust to your audience. If you have a very long runway, you probably can't go more than 8 or 10 feet without doing a turn. Otherwise you will have gone too far past the people viewing you. They wouldn't get a chance to see the front and the back of the garment, so you would vary your turns accordingly.

RUNWAY FORMAT B

ASSIGNMENT

Copy Runway Format B on the blank runway. Again take your pencil, and without lifting it from the paper, follow the numbers. Let the pencil make your turns and you will get that feeling of smoothness so necessary when you're actually modeling on a runway.

Now, do it yourself. Walk over to one of the stairs to enter and practice your Format B.

Runway Format B

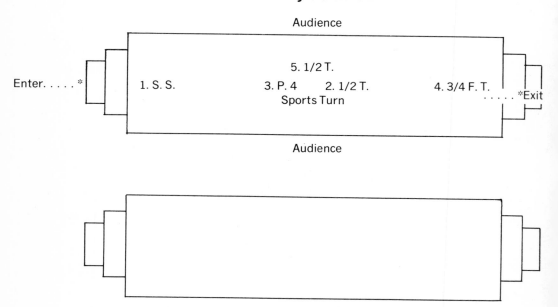

Explanation of Runway Format B

This runway has stairs at the entrance and at the exit. It probably would be the type of runway that is very long. Here you won't have an opportunity to work all the way back again to let the audience see you, so you must work forward.

Let's say you're modeling slacks on the runway. This is how you would do it:

1. Step up on the runway, make a sports stance picture with your slacks and pose for just a split second.

2. Walk briskly down to—or approximately just past—the center of the runway and do a Half Turn.

3. Take four steps with a Pivot Four, and bend knee in a Sports Turn.

4. Walk down to the end of the runway, do a Three-Quarter French Turn (Sports).

5. Walk back to center, make a Half Turn and walk off briskly. You might pause for just a moment for a picture, and off you go.

Note: On 3 and 4, remember this is a Sports Turn and the knee should be bent sharply to show the line.

RUNWAY FORMAT C

ASSIGNMENT

Copy Runway Format C in the blank runway and follow it with your pencil. I like this particular type of runway, where a girl will enter at one end, and the exit steps will be at the center.

Runway Format C

Exit

6. 3/4 F. T.

Entrance

5. E. T. & 1/2   3. 1/2 T.   1. E. T.   4. P. 4   2. 1/2 T.

Audience on all four sides

Explanation of Runway Format C

In this type of runway, the entrance stairs are at one end, and the exit steps are at the center. Actually the steps can be placed anywhere that would furnish a good spot for you to step off and go through the audience a little way to your exit. It makes it easy for you to get back to the dressing room and still gives the audience an opportunity to see a little more of you. The steps will generally be placed on the side that is convenient to the dressing room.

Let's assume you're removing a coat.

1. Enter at the assigned end of the runway, do a European Turn in the center.

2. Walk down to the end and do a Half Turn. At this point, you would have unbuttoned your coat and opened it.

3. As you walk back past the center, you would be removing your coat and—just to fake it a little on the complete removal—do a Half Turn.

4. As you're adjusting the coat—whether you're folding it over your arm or putting it up on your shoulder—finish up on a Pivot Four.

5. You will have enough time to turn again, going back to the end of the runway. Very smoothly, do a European Turn and a Half, which returns you facing the center of the runway.

6. Walk back to the center, reach around with your downstage foot (the one that's nearer the steps) and do a Three-Quarter French Turn. This will place you in a position to walk smoothly down the steps and off.

Note: If you're a little confused about your downstage foot, it would be your foot nearer the steps. Reach around with your downstage foot, and that Three-Quarter French Turn sets you straight to exit down the steps.

T-SHAPE RUNWAY FORMAT D

You could look at this T-Shape strictly as a stage with an extended runway, but look at it as if it were in the middle of a room. This stage has been built in the Plaza Hotel in New York and in other hotels, and it is an excellent format.

So is an X-Shape. Or a V. I saw a fashion show that was quite magnificent. Two models came out from two different entrances, and the runways V'd out from a small stage where the commentator stood. The girls modeled in this V-Shape. They stepped off the ends and walked over to another runway—a small straight one standing independently. Everyone in the room had an opportunity to eventually see all the models.

This gives you a good idea of the different and spectacular ways to set up fashion shows. When you're thinking of organizing a fashion show of your own (which we'll discuss in detail in Chapter 12) you'll use your own ingenuity and ideas as to where to set up your runways. You must have plenty of models when using the T-Shape runway; otherwise you could get into some difficulty.

I recently completed a fashion show for Mobil for an audience of fifteen hundred women. We had three runways; the first one was 30 feet long from the center stage. Then the models walked through the audience about 30 feet to another runway. They stepped off that runway and walked another 20 feet to still another runway. Each runway had to do for about five hundred people.

We had three models coming up on each runway at the same time, so that all of the women could see models simultaneously. Each girl modeled separately while two models posed.

Common sense must be used in trying to do this. We had two dress-

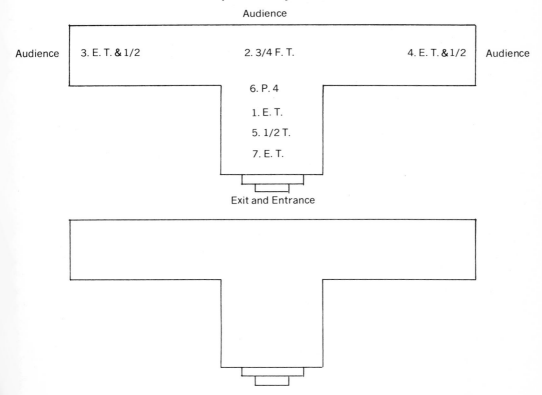

T-Shape Runway Format D

ing rooms backstage, one at either end of the ballroom—one for the girls working at one end and one for the girls working at the other. This was a great production and a most effective way to use three runways.

ASSIGNMENT

Copy your T-Shape Runway Format D on the blank stage. Follow numbers with your pencil.

Note: There are also L-shaped runways, and V-shaped runways. They can be made many different ways. The T-Shape is one of the most popular.

Explanation of T-Shape Runway Format D

Coming back to our T-Shape runway, visualize this in a small T-Shape in your living room, if possible. As you can see, there are steps on one side only.

All right. You're wearing your chiffon formal and you're ready to go on.

1. Walk to the center of the first portion of the runway, and do a European Turn.

2. Walk on down to the center—we're assuming the audience is around you on three sides—and reach around and do a Three-Quarter French Turn. Direction depends on which way you feel you must go first. In this particular case, if you're modeling by yourself, it really wouldn't matter which way you go or come back. It would only be important if you were modeling with a partner.

3. Reach around with the Three-Quarter French Turn, which will place you in position to go to one end of the runway and do a European Turn and a Half, which looks beautiful with a formal.

4. Walk quickly to the other end of the runway and do another European Turn and a Half.

5. Walk to the center and down the runway toward the exit, and three quarters of the way down, do a Half Turn.

6. Take four steps and do a Pivot Four.

7. Come back to the end and do a European Turn before you glide down the stairs. This can be varied, as you can do a Three-Quarter French Turn at either end.

Note: You don't have to do a Three-Quarter Turn on 2. You can just walk over. Also, you could substitute a Three-Quarter French Turn on 3 and 4, and eliminate the Three-Quarter French Turn on 2.

6
GROUP MODELING AND FINALES

Group modeling is being done more often in fashion shows. You may model with two, three, four, five, or six models at the same time. Don't let this confuse you. Just follow the director's instructions. Utilize to advantage all the turns you've learned in this book.

Usually, the girl to your left is the lead model. Keep pace with her. This could vary if a producer or director has a different idea. Learn to follow directions and be adaptable.

By keeping your eye on the lead girl, you may find yourself modeling shoulder to shoulder. You may also model in a line where you will be a lead girl or a follower. In any case, keep your distance as directed and pay full attention to your partner without the audience being aware of it.

You will learn to start your turn as soon as your lead model makes her first move. There will be times when your lead model may actually half-finish a turn before you start yours. You may be requested to wait until your partner completes a turn and then you will do your turn. Learn every way.

Group modeling is very effective in showing colors and designs together. One model may not always tell a fashion story as brilliantly as group modeling.

The more talents you have besides being able to model, the farther you will go in the field. If you can dance well, or have had any ballet, you'll be able to go into elaborate production numbers. Be able to do the new dance steps so that you'll be ready if asked to perform.

There may be a fraction of a moment onstage when you may be asked to swing into a dance step because it will point up the feeling of a costume. An example would be doing a bit of a Charleston for a Roaring 20's dress with fringe.

You'll often see bits like this in a show. You may need a bit of a tango, with black velvet and a red rose. Some of the fashion shows featuring very mod, way-out clothes had the models dancing all the way down the runway. They never *stopped* dancing.

This is an extreme, but a girl who can dance will have advantages in a fashion show. Keep up with your dance steps, and put a little fun in your fashion life!

FORMATS FOR GROUP MODELING

There are many interesting ways for two or more fashion models to show their costumes. Here are a few samples, to give you ideas. Don't be afraid to try any original idea with groups. You may incorporate one or more male models, dancers, or a vocalist. Be as ingenious as you want to be.

Group Format—All Models Onstage

After each girl models and returns to her position, all models change their pose together. The next model in line steps out and models. Poses may all be in the same direction, or different. Each girl models in any manner that's best for her costume.

Group Format—Two Models

One model goes to Center Stage and poses. The second model joins her and poses. They model together, using Format A or B. They will keep approximately 6 feet apart in Format B, with the second model keeping her distance and pace matched to the first model. If Format A is used, they go to opposite corners, crossing over or passing each other when they meet at center. European Turns are done just *after* they pass each other. Keep to the right.

Group Format—Three Models

Models come onstage one at a time and pose. The center girl models by herself in any way she pleases; then back to Center Stage and poses. The two outside models will do a Format C. After the first model completes her first European Turn, the second model will start her modeling. After she has completed the European Turn, the third model will begin; all three pacing themselves to complete in the same manner with their exit.

Group Format—Four Models

A. Walking onstage two at a time, the models pose to fit the staging; 4 to 6 feet apart looks good. A larger stage may require more space. All four do a Pivot Four together, being careful to keep shoulder to shoulder. Have one center girl be the lead girl, and the other models keep with her pace. After returning from a Pivot Four, two models on Stage Left or Right step out and walk closely together, shoulder to shoulder, to the opposite corner of the stage. At this point, one model will be the lead girl, and the other will walk about 6 feet behind her and copy whatever stage format she sets up, or simply do what she does. Take it easy, and simply be her shadow.

B. All models come to the center of the stage and space themselves in an attractive manner. The two center girls walk downstage to the footlights, do a Three-Quarter French Turn, so that each girl will be ready to walk in the opposite direction. Both walk to the opposite corner of the stage and do a European Turn and a Half. Then they walk back to center downstage and turn together to walk upstage and do a Pivot Four. The two outside models follow the same format before exiting. All four exit together. All may go off on one side, or two models may go off on Stage Left and two on Stage Right.

Group Format—Five Models

Five models may enter onstage from different areas—two models from Stage Left, two from Stage Right, and one model walk in from Stage Center. If this isn't practical, have all five walk in from one side and pose in an effective manner, keeping an even distance, or walk in and pose one at a time. The two outside models go to Stage Right, and one model walks to Stage Left. All three do a Three-Quarter French Turn. Go to center and do another Three-Quarter French Turn, which will have the three models with their backs to the audience. Then walk together into a Pivot Four. Walk to your original entrance position and pose. While approaching your position do a European Turn if there is room to do it with ease. The two center models that have been posing will immediately walk to the opposite corners of the stage and do a European Turn. They then walk to Stage Center and pass each other; as they reach Stage Left and Stage Right, respectively, they will each do a Three-Quarter French Turn and start back to their original positions at Stage Center. Just as they reach their positions, all models walk off simultaneously. It is important that the girl who will lead offstage watch the last two models carefully so as to time the exit perfectly. All models may do a European Turn before exiting.

Group modeling is flexible, and don't be afraid to change anything that will improve your staging.

Note: Continuous moving and following through on time make any group modeling more beautiful. Stage Left girl is usually the lead girl. However, any model in front would automatically be the lead girl when working together in a single line.

If there are three or more models working together, Center Stage Left girl would be the lead girl. When you follow a model, keep close observation of your distance. You can see your lead model out of the corner of your eye, without making it noticeable.

Models should have an opportunity to rehearse together before show time. Once a model has worked the formats, rehearsals may not be necessary for future shows.

Now it is your turn to take the model turns you have learned, and incorporate an idea of your own. A handsome male vocalist can be used very well with a show. He may take a model's hand to lead her out of her position. He can sing to her, and assist with coats.

A dancing model can add a great deal of zest to a show, too. She must wear something suitable to dance in.

Working in groups requires some entertainment between showings. This allows the models time to dress and be ready to work together.

If you are fortunate enough to have ten or more models, you may work in groups of five or less and manage very well. This requires professional models who can dress quickly and know what they're doing. Work hard at being the best.

All of these group formats can be adjusted to runway modeling, using the same ideas.

FINALES

At the end of every fashion show, there will be some kind of a finale. This is very important. It's a strange thing, but if something should go wrong with the finale, it leaves a bad taste even though the rest of the show was beautiful. Learn to handle your finales.

In training our students, we think it is wise for them to work with groups on coming out from Stage Left and Stage Right. Use both sides in practice. In school, we will use three girls or more—four, five, six and on up to eight girls—and then they learn to pace themselves to interesting finale groups.

For instance, we'll have three girls. They would be spaced farther apart—one in the center, one on either side. Never in a straight line. Always have one girl farther back or forward, or have them all at a different line, if there are interesting props on the stage.

Semicircle Finale

With a group of six or eight, which makes up an average fashion show, this is the way to do the finale.

Learn to pace yourself approximately 3 to 4 feet from the next model, and your only responsibility lies in keeping an eye on the girl in front of you. If every girl does this, it will be fine. The lead girl knows where she's going to stop, then the second girl will stop approximately at her place, and on down to the third, fourth, fifth, and sixth girl. The first model would be closer to the footlights; the center models would be back farther; and the last models—sixth or eighth, depending on how many you're working with—would be down closer to the footlights, parallel to the first model, to give a semicircle effect.

There are various ways to do this. The models can come out, two on either side and two in the center, or one from Stage Left and one from Stage Right, until all are onstage. There are various basic ways to fill a stage evenly.

It is very effective to do it unevenly, but not to favor one side so that it becomes unbalanced. If there are heavier props on one side, use more models on the other, but there must be an artistic eye—an eye to proportion—on this. In practicing, it's enough to know that you take your pace from the model before you, and know where you're going.

Sometimes the girls do a Three-Quarter French Turn before they stop to pose. This is attractive. Sometimes, as they go off, one girl will do a European Turn just before she exits. You really have to have the feeling that you're doing a finale.

See the diagrams on the following pages. You'll find that the steps are excellent for you to try. In practice, you can see that you need more than one girl. Pacing evenly, three models may come out together. They may come out one at a time or they may come out close together. Usually, models will come out following one another, and this is the way we teach our students to do.

Remember, you may be given instructions for a finale, and may not have the opportunity to practice it. We hope you will, because I

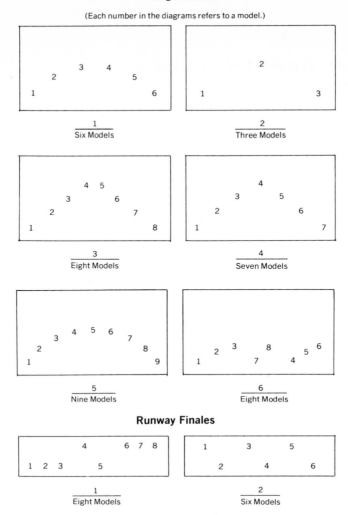

Stage Finales

(Each number in the diagrams refers to a model.)

1
Six Models

2
Three Models

3
Eight Models

4
Seven Models

5
Nine Models

6
Eight Models

Runway Finales

1
Eight Models

2
Six Models

think finales always turn out better if the models have a chance to rehearse. If you can't rehearse your finale, though, a diagram will help. If a diagram is drawn and you can see how you have to go, whom you are to follow, and where your position is onstage, then all you have to do is gauge the distance with your eyes and subtly make adjustments, if necessary.

There are any number of ways to have a sucessful finale. On a runway, you can form a straight line, or make a little zigzag, or center your groups, or have a continuous walk on and off. Many times in a finale on a runway, a model may use a Half Turn once. She'll face one side and another girl will face the other. Then they will do a turn and change with each other, so that the audience on either side will have an opportunity to see all of the girls.

Now, with so many production shows being staged, many clever ideas are utilized. This would, of course, involve following instructions from each director.

FASHION SHOW PICTURES

Here are the finales and some examples of group modeling seen in the "Tropicana Holiday Fiesta" fashion show in the Tropicana Hotel, Las Vegas.

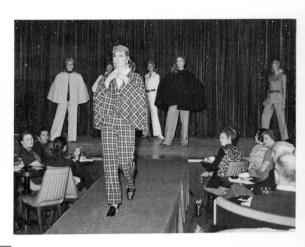

DESIGNER OSCAR DE LA RENTA

A good fashion show will always have one or more models in action and is never slow. This is a typical example of what you may be called upon to do for an opening scene. Posing perfectly onstage with what you are modeling until it is your turn to step out and model as you see the girl in the foreground doing.

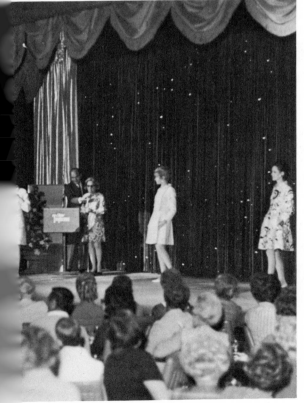

DESIGNER MALCOLM STARR

Three models were used in this scene. The center girl is modeling first while the other two cross over and change places rather slowly to keep a moving background of fashion. As the model reached the end of the runway, the model who was to follow stepped into the spotlight and proceeded with her modeling. Always watch closely when it is your turn, and still do what is expected of you onstage.

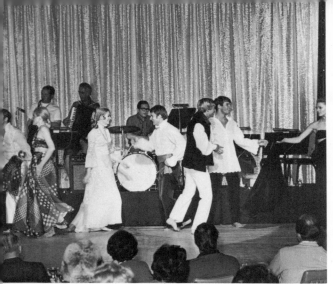

DESIGNER ROYER OF ACAPULCO

We have written about a model being versatile. These fashion models were selected because they were also able to dance. They danced with male models in a lively modern way and used model's turns to the beat of the music. Usually you will dance in your own manner, but having a natural sense of rhythm and beat is most essential. Are you prepared for a dancing scene?

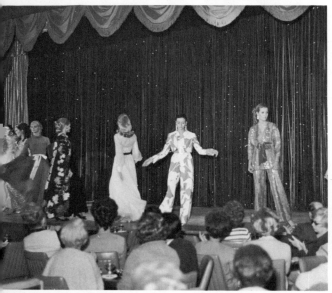

DESIGNER ADELE SIMPSON

You are looking at a stage finale in motion. The models walked quickly onstage and then moved back and forth in their area doing any turns they wanted to in the small space. When the lead model started to exit they all watched the model they were to follow and exited beautifully. You can too!

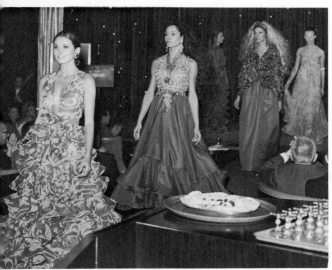

DESIGNER OSCAR DE LA RENTA

Notice the perfect spacing of the models as they walk down the runway and off for the exit in the finale of the show.

7

MODELING JACKETS, COATS, AND ACCESSORIES

MODELING SWEATERS OR SNUG-FITTING JACKETS

There is a special technique to modeling a jacket or sweater, or a coat. The object is to show the audience every angle of the garment —on or off—and every movement must be graceful, continuous, without a break.

Let's assume, then, that you are modeling a jacket. Use your mirror, and follow the suggestions, and the pictures.

Walk out as if onstage, wearing the jacket closed or buttoned. Pose according to what you feel is a good pose for the particular costume. This will vary—depending on length of jacket, sleeve detail, or pockets. Continue forward to downstage and do a Pivot Four.

If there are buttons to open, you will unbutton them as you are walking backstage to complete your Pivot Four. Starting time for unbuttoning will vary depending on the number of buttons you need to work with on your jacket. Make every effort to unbutton your jacket with one hand. Naturally, if the buttons are difficult, use both hands. Notice how the buttonhole is made, and push the button through with the thumb and fingers the easiest way. Once the button has been started through the hole your thumb will push it through with ease. Usually, it is best to start unbuttoning at the bottom and work up to the top. This will leave your hands near the top to ease the jacket (or coat) off the shoulders for removing, or opening, whichever the case may be.

As you turn back, raise your hands gracefully to a comfortable position just above the bust line and gently ease the jacket off your shoulders as you walk toward your audience. (See Picture 14 on "Using Hand Positions," Chapter 3.)

1. This picture, like 2 and 3, shows a back view which is not visible to the audience. When a fabric clings, the back hemline of the jacket may be pulled to make removal easier.

2. As removing a jacket or sweater is not an attractive process to view from the back, when possible the audience should not see it. We will assume that this is a sweater that is tight at the wrist and has to be pulled off. Reach back with one hand and pull the cuff down to your hand.

3. Reach over with the other hand; now you have both cuffs in one hand. At this point, you would be up close to the footlights.

4. Remove one sleeve by pulling your arm out of it. The bare arm is the one that is turned to the audience. The movement is possibly a little strained because we are showing you the back (you must visualize the wall as the audience), but the audience is not seeing this. In the process of turning. . .

5. . . . Your bare arm is turned toward the audience and you have the jacket in front of you. When you are working on runways, make a turn and complete a Pivot Four when removing the jacket. The removal of a jacket should be as graceful as possible without the audience being aware of any difficulty. As the back is being shown to the audience, the commentator can discuss it while you proceed to fold the jacket.

6. This shows what you will do with the jacket now that it's in front of you as you walk back. Place the two cuffs together. . .

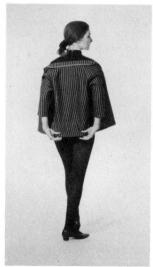

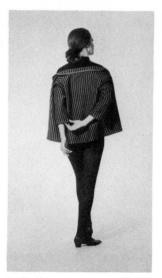

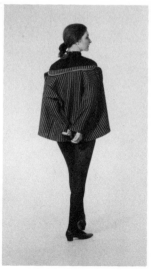

1. Some sweaters or jackets may need a little pull at the back to remove more easily.

2. Pull one sleeve down to hand.

3. Holding cuff in hand, pull other sleeve down to same hand.

4. As you draw arm out of sleeve, turn the bare arm to audience and bring jacket in front of you.

5. With jacket in front of you, continue walking and start final process of removing it.

6. Take both cuffs in free hand as you pull other arm out.

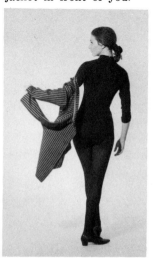

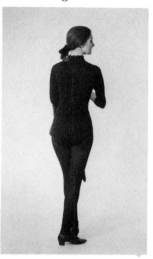

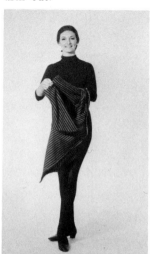

7. . . . and in the other hand take the collar label.

8. You may casually hold your two center fingers in at the label and throw the jacket up onto your shoulder toward the back.

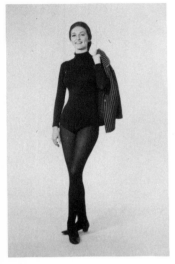

7. Hold jacket at center back.

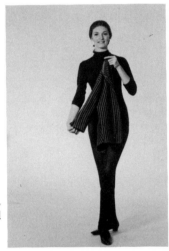

8. Casually lift jacket up on shoulder, holding it with two center fingers and thumb.

Note: It must be emphasized that a model *does not stop* if she takes off a jacket to show a dress. The effect is far prettier if she learns to pace herself so that she doesn't stop in the process.

If she is onstage, she is aware that there is an audience and she can do a great deal to camouflage any unattractive process.

If she is on a runway, she will do a Half Turn at the point where she removes the jacket. As she starts to put it in place over her arm, she'll do another Half Turn. These two Half Turns—doing them in a Pivot Four in the center—will camouflage working with the jacket.

With the particular jacket illustrated, removal is difficult and it has to be pulled off. Always keep moving, no matter how difficult. The model never stops and looks as if she is struggling.

MODELING COATS—TWO VERSIONS

Version 1

You've learned how to remove a jacket or a sweater with tight sleeves. You have to pull it off by the sleeves. There is another way of taking off a coat. Anything that will slide off the arms easily should be removed in this manner. It can be a short jacket or a coat of any length. A very long evening coat would hit the floor. Whether you should allow it to touch the floor or carpet would depend on where the show is held. If it is permissible—and you should ask your coordinator—it's most effective to let a coat drag casually on the carpet. It gives a more nonchalant, almost careless feeling, and can sometimes give more effect to a showing.

Let's look at the pictures and see how our model does it. Follow them closely.

1. Let's suppose you have walked onstage with your coat fully buttoned (if it has buttons) or closed. Your audience must always see the coat as it would be worn when closed. This will determine the cut and line. Are there pockets? What are the details?

2. You will walk downstage as in Format A and, on returning upstage and showing the back of your coat, you will unbutton it, preferably with one hand. Turning around, you will open it. There are many ways of opening a coat. You could open it with your hand on the waist, letting the coat hang straight on one side. You could bring the coat back by having both your hands back at the waist.

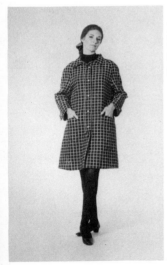

1. Walk onstage with coat closed. Use hands in pockets without ruining line of coat. Note thumbs are out. Hands are not plunged into pockets.

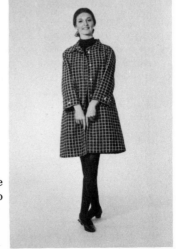

2. Reach with full length of arms to take hold of edge of coat. Hold with thumb and center fingers to open.

3. You may want to show the dress or lining, so you will hold your hands at the edges of the coat and open it to display the lining.

4. Now you start to remove the coat. Lift your hands up to a comfortable position and, using your thumb and two center fingers, drop the coat off your shoulders. Grasp the fabric gracefully so that your hands will not look stiff. Notice how graceful our model's hands are in the picture. Because the coat has enough width in the sleeves, and assuming that you're not wearing anything that would cause the lining to stick — most linings are smooth — the coat literally would drop to the floor if you didn't catch it. At this point, let it drop straight down to your hands. You might possibly have to pull the cuffs a little bit. Notice how our model has lifted her hands to catch the coat at the shoulder line, right in the arms where the sleeves fit in. You'll never drop the coat if you hold it this way. There's a little lift to the elbows, and you catch it right in the shoulder.

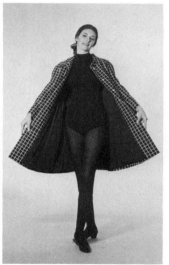 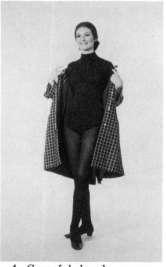 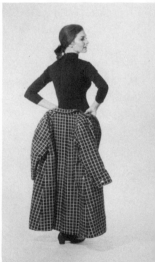

3. Notice how graceful and relaxed hands can look at edge of coat as you open it to show dress and lining of coat.

4. Graceful hands removing coat off shoulders.

5. Lift hands up sharply to catch coat as it falls into hands by shoulders.

5. This is the way the coat should appear from the back. (The audience will not see this.) The coat is not touching the floor, because you've lifted it clear.

6. Now take your hands and move them firmly over to the center of the collar and grasp it there. You started from the shoulders and now you're moving to the center label.

7. When you get both hands together at the label, drop your left hand and hold the coat firmly with your right hand. You've done this while walking toward your audience. They haven't seen it at all. You're down at the footlights at this point, going toward them.

8. As you turn, you will bring the coat in front of you with your right hand.

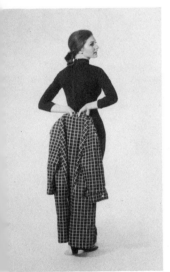

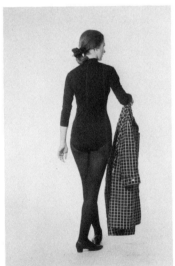

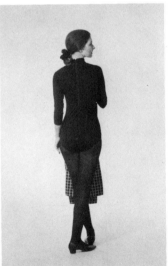

6. Move hands quickly to center label.

7. Hold coat firmly by label and bring it in front of you as you do Half Turn. We show more coat in picture for demonstration.

8. This shows you how the coat can be hidden and worked with while walking upstage.

9. As you walk upstage, the commentator will be talking about the back of your dress. Hold the sleeves together. Your hand is at the label in the center of your collar, so that the coat is perfectly even, and your other arm is extended. The audience does not see this.

10. Fold the sleeve over in front, and wrap your coat over your arm. I mean a nice, full wrap. So many girls cheat on this and have just a little short edge and a long one.

11. The coat can be folded actually in half by being a full length over the arm. At this point, you should be just about ready to turn back to your audience again.

12. Place the coat over at the side of your hip and turn back to the audience. The garment will be low at the hip, not up at the waist. Your hand will be firmly on the seam of the dress to hold the weight of the coat. Your viewers can now see your dress.

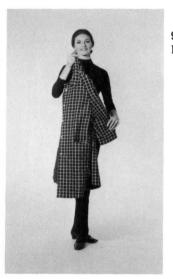

9. Bring coat up and take sleeves in one hand.

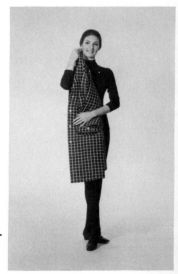

10. Fold sleeves over coat.

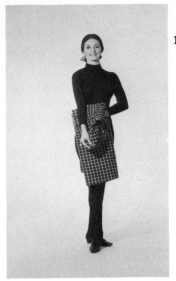

11. Fold coat over in half.

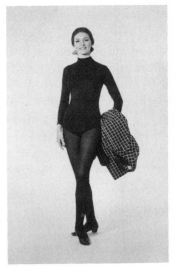

12. Place coat firmly to side of lower hip.

The mistake that so many models make is in holding the coat too high, so that it hides the waistline of the dress. It should always be brought very low, almost resting on the upper thigh.

Now you're ready to walk forward or go over to the other side of the stage. When you're walking toward the side of the stage and the coat is toward the audience, you should remove it and switch it over to the other arm. This is done very easily as you walk. It is something you must practice.

Timing is important. Make your turn, hold the coat at the label and put it up on your shoulder, as we will be showing with a jacket. Study the different ways of removing a coat or jacket and be able to interchange them. There are some coats that look well up on your shoulder, and some that do not.

A coat should stay away from the audience. Once the coat is removed, it's not so important as what is underneath it, which, by this time, the commentator will be describing. If you're walking from Stage Left to Stage Right and find that your coat is over your arm and toward the audience, just casually bring it over the other arm. With a European Turn, naturally part of the coat will be seen, but you'll end up walking and they'll see the dress. It must be performed very easily.

At first, you may find that you'll be too slow, that your coat hasn't dropped sufficiently. It should be hidden at all times. The process of folding would go on while your back is toward your audience. You actually move continually, but quite effortlessly and without rushing, except when the other models would have too long a wait.

Review: Beginning with Picture 4, when you've lifted your arms to remove the coat, you never stop from that point on. Movements are timed so perfectly. When you have caught the coat, as in Picture 7, and have it in one hand, that's when you're ready to turn and bring it in front of you. Remember, the actions in Pictures 7 through 11 are all done when you're walking *away* from your audience.

This way to remove a coat is designed for modeling onstage. If you do not have a stage, it would have to be done the same way on a runway. If you do have a stage, it can be done beautifully, hiding the process of removing and folding as shown in the pictures.

Version 2

There is another way of removing a coat onstage or on a runway. It can be a long or a short coat, but it must be one that can be easily taken off. If at any time you have to *pull* something off, you must go back to the instructions for sweater or jacket removal.

Here is how you would remove a jacket or coat—one that will come off easily and loosely—as you are walking from Stage Left to Stage Right or from Stage Right to Stage Left. The object is to remove it in the process of walking. There could be several reasons for this procedure. You may just want to do it this way, or you may have forgotten to do it at the center, or there may not be room enough for you to remove your coat gracefully in the width of the stage. The coat must always be removed *away from the audience.*

1. Let's imagine that you've just finished a Three-Quarter French Turn at the end of Stage Left. As you walk over to Stage Right, you will take your arm out of the sleeve on the side of the audience, so that they can begin to see the dress underneath. You don't want them to see the jacket or coat coming off.
2. You have slipped your arm out completely and let it fall, and you're still holding the jacket firmly with your upstage hand.
3. Now reach over with your downstage hand to get a grip on the center part of the collar, as much as possible, to get it up to your shoulder and hold it firmly while you slip the arm out.
4. Hold it a moment with both hands.

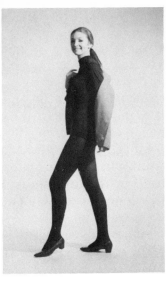

1. Hold coat securely with upstage hand as you slip downstage arm out of coat.

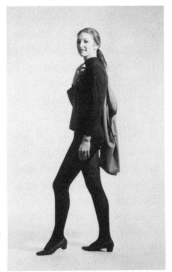

2. Downstage arm is out, and you continue to hold jacket securely with upstage hand.

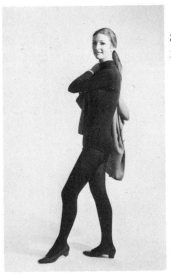

3. Hold coat with downstage hand as you slip upstage arm out of sleeve.

4. You will be holding coat for a moment with both hands as you prepare final adjustment.

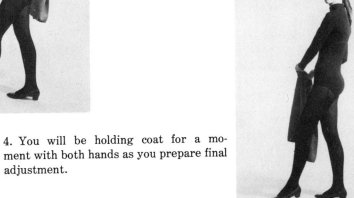

5. If it is a short jacket that you can drop, drop it completely, and simply walk over to the other side of the stage, holding it with your upstage hand.

6. Or you can bring it up onto your shoulder, which would be convenient if you have a long coat and don't want it to touch the floor. You could hold it up, still walking and showing the side of your dress, but for a brief moment you're holding the coat up off the floor with both hands. Then you drop the other arm and the coat will be right up on your shoulder, but you will have to hold it briefly with *both* hands if it's a long coat and you don't want it to touch the floor. If the garment is short, you can drop it completely, as in Picture 5.

You may be in the center of the stage, so you simply do a European Turn. Be careful here. You do a European Turn slowly. You don't want the coat to swing out and look flippant, unless there's a particular reason. For instance, it may be a very lively fashion and you're deliberately aiming for such an effect. Here, again, it is the mood of the costume that determines this.

As you drop the coat, you can go into a European Turn if there's space for it. You may end up at the side of the stage and finish with a Three-Quarter French Turn, but a turn can be done—if it's permissible within your area of staging—if you have your coat up on your shoulder or if you've dropped it.

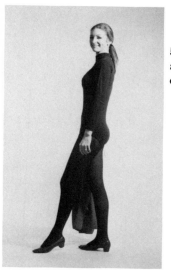

5. You may drop short jacket to side as you continue walking to complete another turn.

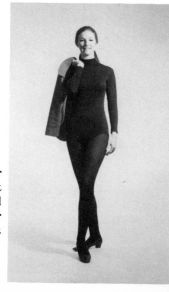

6. If coat or jacket looks well on your shoulder, merely slip it up and hold it by center label with center fingers and thumb again. You may also fold it over arm and place at hip as shown in first version of removing coats.

Removing a Short Jacket

If you're modeling a short jacket, remember, you would always come onstage with it—or a coat—closed, no matter what style or type it is. It must be seen, whether it has buttons or not, as it would look before you open it. Now follow our suggestions through each step.

1. You have modeled forward, we'll assume, and shown the jacket. Now, as you turn around to your audience, you have gracefully opened up one side of the jacket. Remember, you must be aware that the hand remains graceful. Opening the jacket with your thumb and two center fingers, keep your little finger and your forefinger extremely easy and relaxed. (See Picture 11 on "Using Hand Positions," Chapter 3.)

Because it is a short jacket, you can, if you wish, use your hand at the waist or in some other position that will accent the skirt. Or you can just let your hand relax, but opening the jacket to show the lining and the blouse underneath is what we're emphasizing at this point. You may possibly open up both sides of the jacket, using your hands in the same way you would with one hand. (See Pictures 12 and 13 on "Using Hand Positions," Chapter 3.)

2. Slip your jacket from your shoulders as you have in all of our previous coat positions. Because it is a short jacket, though, be sure you do it as we show it in our sweater and jacket illustrations in this chapter. Take hold of the jacket at the back and pull it down, especially if you're wearing a sweater or blouse that might cling to it. You have to give a little pull at the back edge of your jacket. Let it fall down into your hands, catching it at the armholes and shoulder top.

At this point refer back to the instructions in this chapter on removing a coat and follow them. Version 2 will explain how to handle a short jacket for the final picture onstage. Because there is less work involved with a short jacket that slips off easily you may accomplish removing it during a European Turn. Practice continuity and continuous motion.

Note: Here is something you must watch out for: When you do a European Turn, don't fling the jacket too far away from the body or flip it out. Do your turns slowly and smoothly, so that the jacket will stay in close to the body, unless, again, the feeling of the costume will allow you to be flippant while showing it. It depends on the mood and feeling of the costume.

Removing a Cape

You will model a cape just as effectively as you've learned to model coats and jackets.

Lift your hand up to one side and hold your cape gracefully but firmly near the collar. Take the other hand and drop the cape off one shoulder. Using the other arm, bring the cape over and hold it momentarily with your hand at the collar, while you bring your inner arm up under the cape near the label to hold it in place. It's just a matter of taking one hand and holding the collar, while you adjust with the other hand to hold it permanently.

If it is a short cape, you could drop it or bring it up to your shoulder as in Pictures 5 and 6 in Version 2 of "Modeling Coats." You will treat a full-length cape as a full-length coat. It's up to you to experiment with whatever would be most effective.

Note: Usually, capes look very graceful just thrown casually over the shoulder to show the sweeping lines of the design, even when you're showing the dress underneath. You can do both, but the above suggestions show you mainly how to remove the cape, since, in most cases, you cannot drop it as you would a coat.

Handling a Stole

Nothing can look as lovely as a flowing chiffon stole, and there are few things that can look as clumsy and ungainly as one that is handled the wrong way. Get it right in the beginning.

I'd suggest that a serious student buy some inexpensive rayon chiffon. A three-yard length, like the one our model is using, would be just about right. Buy this yardage, or sew together enough old chiffon scarves until they add up to three yards in length, so that you'll get the feel of a stole.

The one we show here is a full-length chiffon stole that we made for practice in the studio. It's extremely awkward to work with, but it really makes a girl use her hands gracefully and become aware of what a stole can do, both for beauty and for the opposite! Look at our two pictures. They tell you which is the right way and which is the wrong way. Practice, and learn.

1. This picture combines all the things you should avoid in handling a stole.

You should not have it clinging around your neck.

Don't let your arms and hands dangle carelessly so that the stole looks like a rag over your shoulders.

Don't let the two hems hang unevenly at the bottom. You can see the difference.

2. To handle this correctly, drape the stole over your shoulders, away from your neck. It will usually feel rather firm about the shoulders, and it should frame your face as would a stand-up collar. If you are going to open the stole, keep your fingers delicately long and, using your thumb and second finger, open it gracefully, keeping your arms extended.

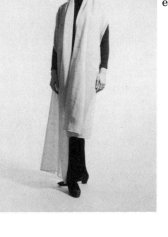

1. Wrong way. Never allow stole to cling to neck. Check that bottom edges are even.

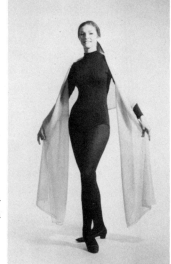

2. Right way. Off the neck, and even hemlines. Graceful hands. Move, and open stole gracefully.

Note: There are various points at which a stole can be dropped. You can drop it at the bend of the elbow and let it fall down to your waist in back, or you can slip it off one shoulder and fold it in half.

Modeling with Handbags and Gloves

HANDBAGS AND TOTE BAGS

Basically, a model will work with a general handbag, a tote bag, and an evening bag. When there are variations in handles, or fresh fashion ideas are introduced, you have to adjust to them and show them the way they should be worn, the way their designers intended them to be.

Our model is carrying a handbag with a handle. There are three ways she would do this. Look at the three pictures and learn the three techniques.

1. The model is working with an average small-size handbag. Use one like it and, holding it with your right hand, place it directly in front of you with the front facing forward. Take your left hand and place it through the handle from the back of the bag, slipping it right onto your arm. You will have it placed as our model has it in this photograph. The front of the bag is displayed more closely to the audience. If you have a bag with front detail that you want the audience to see immediately, this is the way you would carry it. This is important.

2. After you remove the bag from your arm, place it again in front of you, this time turn it slightly to the left (you are holding the bag in

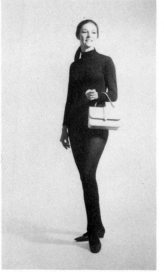

1. Front view of bag.

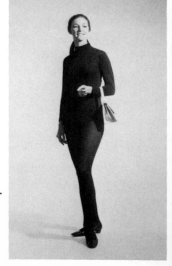

2. To show more front view of costume. Side view of bag.

your right hand) and place your left hand in through the strap from the front of your bag. Your bag will now be to the side, revealing much more of the dress and a side silhouette of the bag. There are times when it is better to model a bag this way. More of the costume is shown, or if you're walking with your side to the audience, the bag is seen by the audience. Always be conscious of the proper placement of the bag.

3. This is the way your arms should look when you drop a bag to the side. One of the most common flaws I find in the practice of this technique is for a girl to bend her elbow as if she's holding a bomb or something equally dangerous! Let the arm relax completely at your side, and let the bag fall very easily and gracefully down by the legs.

Note: Picture 3 also illustrates the way you would carry a tote bag. If you're working with any large bag or a tote bag, you do not put it on your arm. You carry it like this, switching it from one hand to the other. Some of your little chain bags are dropped casually to the side.

Review: These are the three ways you will hold a bag in modeling. Learn to change arms. Drop the bag, don't whirl it. Notice also, in Picture 3, the way our model has her first finger on the strap. This will control your bag. If you should do this while walking and doing a European Turn, your bag will be in control.

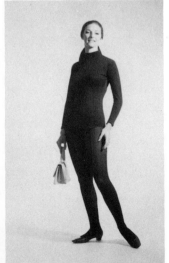

3. Keep arm straight and relaxed. Control with finger on turns, and keep close to body.

EVENING BAGS AND SMALL CLUTCH BAGS

A model must learn to carry an evening bag with ease and grace. The placement of the fingers is important. Whether at the bottom of the bag or at the top of it, your fingers lie long and slim on it. See the photographs and, following them closely, practice with your own small bag.

1. Holding your bag gently, be sure not to clutch it with all four fingers. Usually the forefinger will rest on it lightly at a sloping angle, as you see here. You may bend your elbow slightly and show the bag on the leg a little bit.

2. Simply relax your arm to the side, letting it fall easily and gracefully down the seam of your dress.

3. You may, if you like, bring the bag up gracefully, somewhat in a manner of hugging it to your shoulder. This might be suitable with a small clutch bag if you wanted to get it away from the folds of a dress. Another way to handle this would be to place it behind you as you turn around.

Review: Remember—it may be called a "clutch" bag, but that is the one thing you don't do to it!

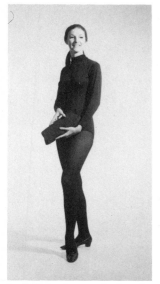 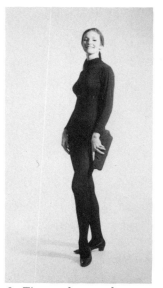 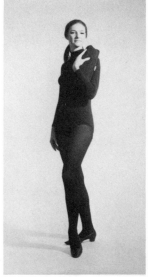

1. Side view of hands, show bag to audience at an angle.

2. Fingers long and graceful along top or bottom of bag. Relaxed against side.

3. Lifted gracefully, and show slim side of hand at edge of bag.

GLOVES

You will notice many different ways in which a model will handle gloves. The main thing to remember is that if you are onstage and the gloves are new, you model them with the fingers to the front so it's obvious that they are gloves. The fingers will be new and they will look all right. Once the gloves have been worn — that is, if they're yours and you're just holding them to give the costume a complete look — it's wise to put the cuffs toward the front. Once gloves have been worn, the fingers get a little out of shape and aren't as attractive. If you hide the fingers, the gloves can be used in this manner.

If you're being photographed for a picture layout, it may be that the gloves are very attractive in the wrist area, so you would carry them with the cuffs foremost. Actually, they can be held both ways.

The important thing is to carry gloves gracefully, using your thumb and center fingers and letting your forefinger flow smoothly along on your gloves, and moving the gloves from one hand to another when you're modeling or doing your turns.

Modeling Hats

Be aware of the different seasons. Pick up any fashion magazine and notice how a girl holds her head in modeling a hat. She will tilt it

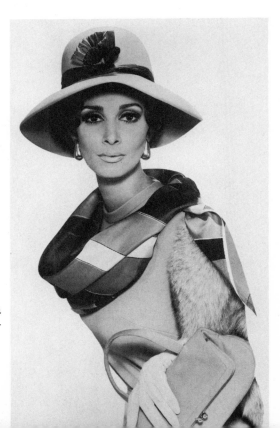

Stunning Wilhelmina modeling a Mr. John hat; notice the graceful way she holds the handbag.

to the side to show the crown. In most cases, she will drop her head forward a little so that the crown will show.

If you were modeling a hat to an audience, you would do the same thing. Tilt your head down a little, and bring it up as you turn your back to the audience. You might lift your chin to show the crown, then very gently turn your head and show the other side.

It is a circling of the head, lifting the chin up when you're away from the audience and dropping it when you're facing them, so that the crown can be shown.

Study the models in the magazines and be aware of how they are photographed in next season's hat styles.

Modeling Jewelry

With jewelry, the same suggestion applies. Look in the magazines and notice how the models display their jewels. Always show the side of your hand, to show beautiful long fingernails and smooth,

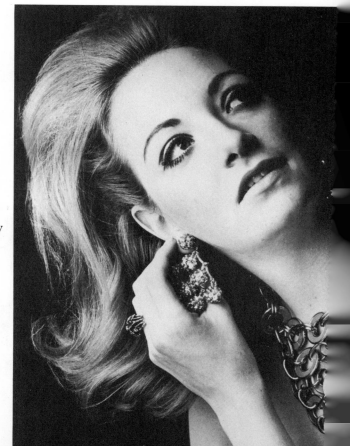

Christie Renee effectively modeling jewelry pieces.

supple hands. The camera reveals every little flaw, but a good trick
is to rub the veins down on the back of the hands as you hold them high
in the air so that veins will not show. Learn to use your hands gracefully, showing the thumb or the little finger to the camera in most
cases.

If you have extremely beautiful hands, you could direct the broad
back of your whole hand to the camera and it wouldn't matter but,
for practical purposes, a three-quarter-to-a-side view is always more
flattering. Place the hand across the body so that you can show a brace-
let, a ring, and earrings all at the same time. The hand will be placed
up near the face and close to an ear, and you can show three pieces of
jewelry in one picture. It's a good way for a client to get more mileage
out of a sitting, too.

Onstage, if you're working with jewelry such as a long string of
beads, you would use your hands very gracefully, touching the necklace with center fingers and thumb.

Here is Christie Renee of the Connecticut Model Agency, Stamford, Connecticut, showing three items of jewelry in one picture. The
hand is soft, smooth, and turned just enough to photograph beautifully, as well as to show all three pieces of jewelry to advantage.

Modeling Furs

You must create a very definite feeling and mood for furs. Furs
are luxury, wealth, the high life, everything wonderful. Even love.
Furs are cuddled, and touched only lightly. You rarely put your hands
in the pockets of a fur coat. They should not bulge. In some instances,
your designer may want you to do this, but he will tell you what his
wishes are. You will manage the collar, and move and adjust it to the
way the coat should be shown.

The inner lining of the coat is only shown if the designer tells you
he wants this. Otherwise, the coat is left closed completely, or occasionally dropped slightly off the shoulder if it looks best this way. As
with any fur, you have to play with it and see which way it looks its
loveliest. Use your hands beautifully, look sophisticated, and as if
you belong to your fur, or it belongs to you!

8
MODELING ASSIGNMENTS

FASHION PHOTOGRAPHY

Almost invariably, the first thing one visualizes on hearing the word "model" is a magazine—complete with glamorous cover girl and bevies of exotic beauties populating the inner pages. Because of this practically universal association of ideas, I'll go into fashion photography first.

WHY PHOTOGRAPHY IS SO IMPORTANT IN THE WORLD OF FASHION

The old cliché of "one picture is worth a thousand words" sums up exactly why a photograph has more of an impact than any written page. A product has to be shown to literally millions of people if it is to sell in volume. That's why magazines, newspapers, billboards, television, and other visual media have photographs, and these photographs must make the reader stop and take a second look. Women depend on fashion magazines to show them the styles for the coming seasons. They will pore over the pictures and look several times before they decide what, to them, is a selling item, or they may take only one look and be sold. This means that you need models, merchandise, and a good photographer. Statistics have proved that any man-made product sells better when a live model is introduced into the photograph. And remember, the pictures you are looking at today in your fashion magazines give you ideas about buying for the next season ahead.

WHERE AND HOW PHOTOGRAPHY IS USED

Photography is used wherever one wants to make a dramatic visual impact. Magazines, newspapers, television, billboards, commercial films. It's used in promotional work and publicity, at trade shows in press kits, and don't forget how important it is for a model to have personal photographs for her portfolio and her agency's headsheets.

How is fashion photography used? To sell a fashion idea, record a style change, highlight a new color, illustrate a new line. It is used editorially in magazines, newspapers, and catalogs, but always it is used to illustrate an idea, make a point, and, finally, to sell a product.

HOW THE MODEL FITS INTO THE PICTURE

When a beautiful model can sell you on the idea that she is in love with the product she's photographed with or in, this helps to sell *you*. I often think there really isn't a complete answer as to why this is. Possibly we identify with a living model. We know we are sold more on an item when a friend recommends it, so when we see a model recommending it, it helps to sell us in the same way.

Whatever the subconscious reasoning, the model is an integral part of photography and fashion. She is a *proven* factor in better sales. How many people take a second look at a dress on a hanger in a window? Very few, compared to the dress that is perfectly draped on a mannequin. Bring that mannequin to life, and everyone is more enthused about the dress. Live models bring the product to life, too, in photography.

STUDIO ASSIGNMENTS

Studios usually are big, bare rooms loaded with equipment. A photographer need not have a glamorous studio. Some photographers do and some don't, but the important thing is that the photographer have the best equipment and a talent to use that equipment and bring to life what his assignment dictates is to be sold.

A model will usually arrive for her assignment completely made up, and then adjust to changes when she is in the studio. The model generally knows in advance what the assignment is, and she is prepared for it. This means the proper accessories, hairpieces, makeup extras, shoes, and undergarments. If she is clever, she arrives somewhat ahead of the scheduled time.

Studios need space for lighting equipment. They usually have backdrops in various shades of paper that can be rolled down from a very high ceiling. The basic shades are blue, black, white, beige, and gray. Other, more dramatic, colors are often included. The background color will be important. The photographer will have many different props, and special props are built for some fashion photographs.

Indoor photographs usually need only the model and a good background paper. After all, it is the costume that is to be featured. It's being sold on a live model.

It is up to the model to know the selling points, and up to the photographer to have ideas. There is a rapport between them if they are both artists at the job. What a joy it is to see a model and a photographer work together when both are experts at their respective professions!

The model learns to move in the confined space of a studio. This is the primary difference from a location assignment. The next major difference is that the model often will have no props or background to assist her with a mood or selling point. She must create this herself, with the help of the stylist and the photographer. Another thing a model must expect in a studio that she probably won't find on location is the hot lights. This is one area in which patience is definitely a virtue, and the ability to react quickly is a positive gain.

LOCATION ASSIGNMENTS

These are—in almost all cases—exciting moments in a model's career. She has an opportunity to travel to many countries so that the photographer can shoot pictures of the fashions against an outdoor or foreign background. The place must be selected to fit the mood and design of the clothes to be shown.

On the other hand, the assignment may not always be easy or comfortable. When you see the model against the background of a majestic mountainside, remember she had to get up there! And she had to arrive there cool, collected, clean, and relaxed looking. Sometimes the weather is very hot, sometimes very cold, but that isn't important. All that matters is an excellent picture. That's all the photographer is interested in.

A whole book could be written on the experiences of models on location photography assignments.

Be prepared with everything you may need for hair, nails, bathing, and personal care. You may not have any assistance on location. On the other hand, a location assignment may take you to a nearby park, beach, waterfront, or public building. Anything that is other than a photographer's studio, outdoors or indoors, is considered a location assignment.

Now that you know a little bit about fashion photography in general, let's go into the specifics and what you'll need for a career in the field.

Basic Camera Poses and Techniques

BODY POSITION

Your posture must be perfect but relaxed, as we have discussed in Chapter 3.

Stand in front of the camera with your body approximately at a three-quarter angle to the camera. Stand with both feet side by side. A three-quarter view of the body is more slenderizing. If, however, you are the slim ten- to twenty-pound underweight fashion model type, you really needn't worry about presenting a three-quarter view to the camera. Nevertheless, please start learning by beginning with this position.

FOOT POSITIONS

Placing all of your weight on the back foot, pick up your downstage foot and point it straight to the camera. You will be in a model's stance. Your weight will be felt in upper thigh and flexed knee. Now imagine your downstage foot is the large hand of a clock, and you are now pointing to twelve o'clock.

1. Downstage toe pointing to twelve o'clock. Raise heel slightly off floor. Keep your knees slightly flexed.
2. Point your toe to one o'clock.
3. Point your toe to two o'clock.

1. Downstage foot to twelve o'clock position.

2. One o'clock position.

3. Two o'clock position.

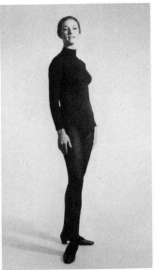
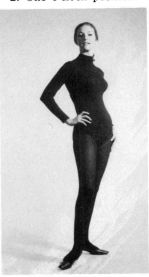
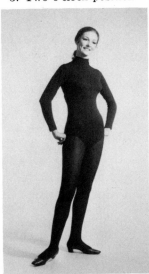

4. Point your toe to three o'clock.
5. Point your toe to four o'clock.
6, 7. Cross over and keep toe to camera.

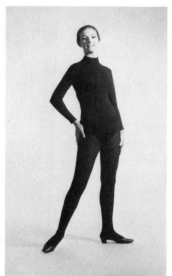

4. Three o'clock position.

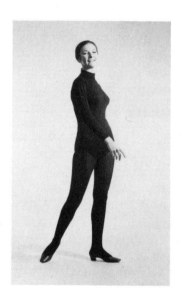

5. Four o'clock position.

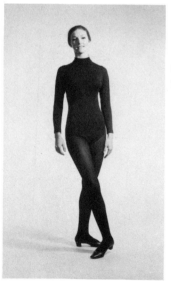

6. Avoid extreme pointing out or in of toe.

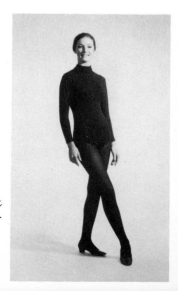

7. See how much better the leg and foot appear when heel is hidden and toe pointed straight to camera.

Your back foot stays at the 45-degree angle and weight remains on your back foot, moving the downstage foot to the various positions and any in-between points to which you are directed. Try to keep the heel of the front foot hidden. This means that you will be aware of pointing your knee to the camera as well. You want the longest, slimmest line to be photographed. The toe will be slightly pointed out, with a consciousness of bringing your heel into or pointing to the back heel. This is necessary to hide the heel. Your photographer may direct you to move inches left, right, back, or forward. Please listen, and do what he asks of you immediately. Change positions on your own — create a mood — pose by yourself.

Note: There are hundreds of different foot positions to study as illustrated by models in the fashion magazines. Make a scrapbook of them and learn to change into at least twelve different types to suit what you are modeling. Remember, props make a difference. You may be on a cliff, lifting a foot upon an object, or in any number of different scenes. Learn to be adaptable.

SHOULDERS

Shoulders should not be squared to the camera. This could give you a football-shoulders look. If you are doing sufficient inner lift, in your body, your shoulders will automatically be down, back, and relaxed. Now, think, "My upstage shoulder should be a bit more relaxed." You will feel the very slightest pull on the side of the neck. This will give your neck a longer and slimmer appearance. Make certain that the front shoulder does not tense or raise. It is just thinking this fraction-lower shoulder that does the trick. With this secret, you increase the effect of a beautiful long, slim neck, and the gently sloping shoulder line and flow will photograph well. Feel it and mirror-check it.

Another trick is to swing the shoulder that corresponds with your downstage foot back and down to give a twist to the fabric of the gown. Motion in fabric is often needed. Practice twisting the other shoulder back slightly; it may be a good position. Practice and compare effects in front of a mirror.

ARMS

Do not let your arms cross in front of your body. It cuts you exactly in half. When you are wearing a costume with sleeves, make certain that your arms are positioned so that they will not obscure the body line in the bust or waist area. When the sleeves and body of the costume are of the same fabric and color, the arms and body become one indistinguishable mass unless there is space between them. The photographer sees to it that the line and fit of the garment are displayed.

When you are wearing a costume that leaves your arms bare, the difference in the color and texture of the skin makes it possible for arm positioning closer to the body, if desired.

Always avoid sharp angles at the elbows, unless directed to do so. Do not let the elbows lie concave into the waist.

If your forearms show, make certain that part of your upper arms shows to the camera's eye so that your forearms do not appear to be growing out of some strange part of your body!

After positioning your arms, turn the elbows back and away from the camera's eye. This will soften or round sharp elbows.

HANDS

Always show the slimmest possible view of the hands to the camera. Relax the hands by doing a few simple exercises before working. Refer to the hand exercises in Chapter 3.

Think of the thumb or the little finger toward the camera. The front part of lovely fingers separated slightly looks well toward the camera also. Avoid exposing the palm or the complete back of the hand to the camera, unless directed by the photographer. Touch any prop with grace, and show a side view of the hand. In most cases, touch the prop with the thumb and center fingers when actually holding the item. The fingers should not appear glued together. They should be slightly separated (the two center fingers lower) for a prettier effect.

Use the hand positions you have learned in Chapter 3. Adjust and smooth your costume gracefully with your hands, touching some items or fabrics with a love or a gentleness, as you would caress fur or velvet.

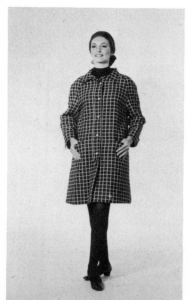

Thumb in pocket and four fingers curled gracefully on fabric. Elbows back and relaxed into body.

POCKETS

Unless directed differently, never plunge your hands completely into a pocket. Place the thumb in the pocket and expose the four fingers gracefully on the outside of the pocket, as pictured. Review Chapter 7, page 87 and you will see the model placing four fingers in the pocket with the thumb exposed. Be certain that the garment is not pulled down or out of shape in any way. Keep the hand close to the body and the elbows back. Watch closely that the costume stays in line. Test both ways for hands, and then do which looks best. The pockets could be placed too high or too low to do either.

ACCESSORIES

When holding an accessory, try to present its longest and slimmest line to the camera, plus, again, the longest and slimmest view of the hand holding it. Generally, the item is held from the bottom, but this is not always true.

Study Chapter 7 carefully on "Modeling Accessories." Look through your magazines and become aware of how the experts model accessories. Practice in front of the mirror doing the same things you see in the magazines.

HEAD

The back part of the top of the head should always be in the tallest position. The chin should be parallel with the floor. This will prevent an undesirable forward or backward tipping of the head or body, which distorts you in the camera's eye. Lower and lift the chin according to the photographer's directions.

A few practice shots with your own camera will reveal good and poor positions of your head. I do not advise you to tell a photographer you have a good side or a bad side! He usually isn't interested, and can judge for himself. Most models are too self-critical. Remember, we are trying to sell a fashion, and you can't be that bad-looking if you have been selected for the job.

Once you are in a position and ready for a head placement, here are a few things to think about:

1. Head held high, chin level with the floor.
2. Turn the head to line up in a straight line with the left hand.
3. Turn the head to line up in a straight line with the right hand.
4. Look straight into the camera lens.
5. Tilt your head one-quarter inch to one side, then to the other side.
6. Tilt the chin down one-half inch.
7. Tilt the chin up one-half inch.
8. Relax those neck muscles.

BATHING SUITS

When sitting down in a bathing suit or tight slacks, remember the following rules:

Never let the weight of the body rest on the thigh close to the camera. It creates a bulge. Sit on a hidden book to take the weight of the body from the thigh, as shown in Pictures 1 and 2. In Picture 3 you see the wrong way to sit.

Never let a foot or ankle look as though it were growing out of a strange part of the body, because no outline of the leg is showing. See Pictures 3, 4, and 5. Lean the weight of the body and limbs away from the camera.

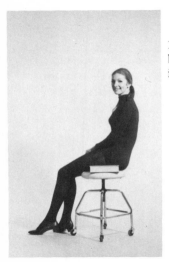

1. This shows where to place the book to take pressure off the thighs in front.

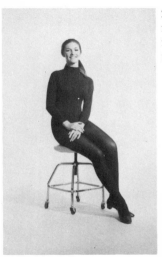

2. Notice there is not a bulge of front thigh on stool as book is taking pressure off front leg. Model is sitting in graceful line.

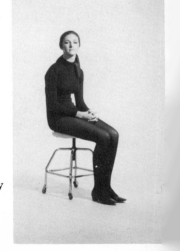

3. Wrong way to sit for photography or any place.

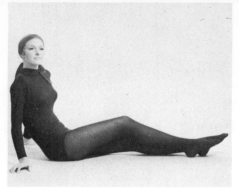

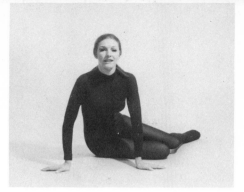

4. Lean away from camera to take pressure off hands, thigh, derriere; flex the elbow joint and raise one knee higher.

5. When leaning into camera keep pressure off front of hands. Soft, flexed elbows. Feet away from camera will make them appear smaller.

UMBRELLA

An umbrella is often used in fashion shows as well as in photography. As you look at fashion magazines note the various ways that models hold umbrellas and other props. Line is very important for excellent composition in photography. Train your eye to see it.

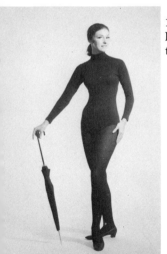

1. Line umbrella up with upstage leg. Keep your hand graceful on the handle.

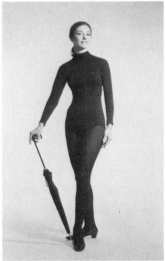

2. Touch umbrella to downstage foot. Note it's same line as arm and hand holding it.

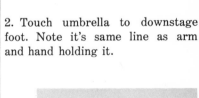

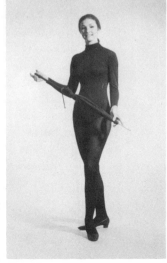

3. If you hold umbrella up with both hands, hold it at an angle and show sides of hands.

Ready for the Camera? A Quick Check

When you are working in front of a camera, it is difficult to remain aware of all the important points simultaneously. It will help if you use a "quick-check" counting method to cover each point until it becomes automatic, and you can then forget the technique, and just animate, assuming you have become familiar with the costume to be photographed. You have experimented with different hand positions in front of the mirror prior to stepping in front of the camera.

CHECK POINTS

1. Stand in a three-quarter view to the camera, with your weight on the back foot. Start moving the front foot to various points.
2. Place your hands in a good position.
3. Line up your chin and head in a good line.
4. Look — and think — the expression you want to achieve.

All of this is accomplished in split seconds and changed into another pose, one right after the other. You learn to move and pose, move and pose. Enjoy yourself and cooperate with the photographer.

Your Responsibility as a Fashion Photographer's Model

1. Be fifteen minutes earlier than your appointment time.
2. Show your best sense of humor — and keep it.
3. Cooperate. If you feel misunderstood, be honest, be tactful, keep conversation light.
4. Do not let anything the photographer says hurt your feelings. He is an individual — an artist — and you are there to work. Not to change him.
5. Have only one objective. Work to produce a good picture. Have confidence in your photographer.
6. Look at yourself as a product. Be warm, but professional.
7. Arrive with sufficient accessories. (Ask, if in doubt.) Be impeccably groomed. Have everything neat and ready for the camera — nails, feet, hair, makeup, accessories. Remember, the camera is very critical and will magnify anything you've neglected.
8. Let your photographer feel important. Voice compliments that you sincerely feel about his work. There must be a rapport between you for the best results. Never question any direction he gives you. A professional photographer knows what he wants.
9. Don't forget! Clean up after yourself before leaving.

Note: These are basic rules. Learn them and then copy the unusual from current fashion magazines, and you will find yourself glowing in front of a camera.

A Modern Approach to Fashion Photography

During the 1968 Modeling Association of America Convention, which was held at the Waldorf Astoria Hotel in New York, I had the pleasure of meeting Tom Jungman of that city. Mr. Jungman is a photographer who has worked out a system whereby fashion models can learn to move in front of a camera. He conducted a workshop demonstrating the principles, and later we were able to take lessons.

As I have instructed you in the previous section, I feel that it is very important for every model to learn basic photography poses so that she knows her own body and face well enough to show her best before a camera. If you have the attributes to become a fashion photographer's model, you should learn more than the basics. You must learn to move with ease and understanding. This is what Mr. Jungman said to me in a letter:

"I've been working with models from all the big agencies in New York, and I was very surprised to find that a majority of them lack the understanding and knowledge of the principles of movement. Any model will make herself more competitive if she has the background in the area of kinesthetics."

I would like to tell you something about the system, so that you can have a better perspective and understanding of it. Then look closely at the pictures in this chapter. You will see what Mr. Jungman means, and why he calls it "Movement in Action."

As Mr. Jungman puts it:

"Whenever you think of movement, generally you think of dancing. Dancing, undoubtedly, is the best-known type of movement, but in the whole area of movement, dancing is only a small part of it. For example, we have movement in all sorts of sports, various forms of self-defense, numerous types of physical exercise, religious ceremonies, performing arts like drama and pantomime, acrobatics and the countless forms of physical works we perform every day."

So when Mr. Jungman talks about movement, he means human locomotion, anything that a person does with his body. In his own words:

"As the name implies, the system is designed to employ movements by the model for a specific purpose, namely, for commercial photography. In photography movement for commercial use, three things are involved: *(1) Technical limitations of photography, (2) Merchandising, and (3) Kinesthetics.* To put this into more practical terms, the model who is commissioned to do a job has to work in a limited space, has to make the merchandise she is wearing or is involved with look attractive and appealing, and in so doing, it is required of her to create an effective body design or a beautiful movement.

"'Movement in Action' is a framework constructed and based on the requirements we have just mentioned. Within this framework, the model is free to create, improvise, and execute her movements to achieve the desired result. She is—in her own right—both a choreographer and a model. I might add here that the day when a model has to depend totally on the photographer's direction for movement is over; now she has to do her own thing. The battle is still going on, however, for the model to free herself from being a puppet-like creature to be transcended into a creative person. Modeling can exist independently on its own creative potential. In order to make it work, the model has to understand the difference between actual movement and photographic movement. In actual movement, there is a beginning and an end, and motion in between. The actual movement has a time sequence, whereas the movement being photographed must be seized in a split second, at a point where the intensity and climax of that movement can be conveyed graphically. The decisive moment to photograph a movement is not at its peak, but rather *at a point before it reaches* its climax. If the climax of an actual movement is recorded, the resulting photograph will be lifeless and static."

According to Mr. Jungman's system:

"The movement performed by the model for the camera is psychophysical. The mind and the body must work together. The mind must control all the parts of the body and their movements and their placements. If the movement is interrupted or the body is rearranged by the photographer, its control must be regained by the model as soon as possible. Every movement performed by the model must have its direction, and all movements executed by the model must be simul-

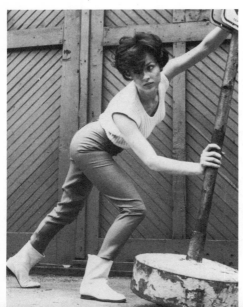

One of Tom Jungman's most brilliant students, Carol Le Feure has a natural instinct for his unique system of "Movement in Action." Part of the course involves work with static props, which are later removed and just imagined. Prop No. 1 is a pole, and the exercise is to establish direction of movement, utilizing various movements of the body. The action is psychophysical; when there is no pole, the mind is creating an imaginary one. In this picture, the pole happens to be physical as well, represented by the stanchion used as a prop.

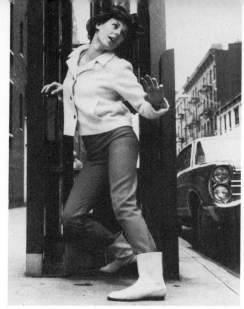

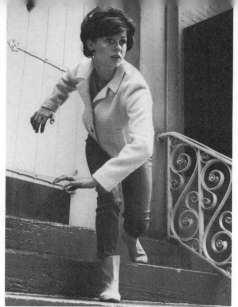

This photograph illustrates the "force of containment" idea, which involves working within a certain defined area or working against a background which would tend to overshadow the model. When working with a group of models, it will determine which one will dominate the group.

The system itself is not creating new movement, but rather incorporating natural movement into an organized design. Everyone has a natural feeling of movement. The system can bring out the natural quality in a model, and give her a framework and direction to analyze, organize, and create her own movement. This picture illustrates that principle.

A photographic exercise in terms of movement: this is what we've been leading up to all along. It is movement and body design in action, and a practical application of Mr. Jungman's system in actual photo assignments or on location. In short, the combination of a theoretical approach and actual exercises to create a practical solution so that you can interpret the mood through movement.

There is generally variation of direction in a movement, a major direction and lesser ones. The major direction here is forward, in contrast to the other parts of the body.

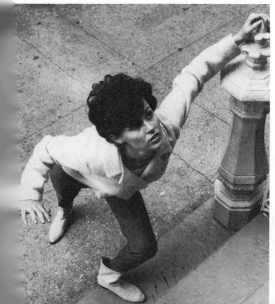

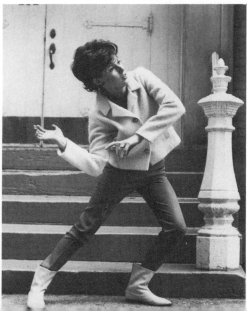

taneous. The model will have complete control of her body in a limited space and can hold a pose naturally for a long time without getting stiff."

One of the *first* things you will learn is how to move parts of the body separately: head, shoulders, arms, torso, waist, and legs. The *second:* to establish a direction of movement. You may use a stationary pole, table, floor, or anything that you can act upon. *Third:* to localize the point of interest which is suggested by the photographer, and then learn to re-establish it and improvise to provide more variation of movement. It is the "Movement in Action" that gives life to the photograph. There are types of positions that a model will learn about as she goes along with this system.

It is understandable why Mr. Jungman calls his studio in New York Models' Workshop. It is also understandable why some models forge ahead of others by being eager to accept and prepare themselves for future photography needs.

One last note. After practicing your basic poses in front of a mirror, you will graduate away from looking at yourself. No mirrors are used, and music isn't needed with this system. In fact, they are forbidden. See how much there is to learn? Working in front of a camera is both a challenge and holds much excitement for the girl who wants to work at it. Let your imagination grow, grow, grow!

Example: Let's imagine you see a beautiful rose which you are to reach out and touch. You take a step forward, reach with the hand gracefully to gently touch the head of the flower, using a complete, graceful body-to-fingertip motion. The photographer tells you to stop just as you reach the flower. You will then go back with your body and your hand to the beginning point and re-establish the idea you started with.

Keep repeating this within a reasonably smooth, slow motion until the photographer lets you know he is satisfied with the pictures he has taken. This may take any number of repeats, from three to forty times. Notice that you have an imaginary point of interest you are going to in your posing. The picture will be taken somewhere between the beginning and the end, *never* at the static stopping point.

Let your own natural movements be used. Let your imagination be magnified. Most of all, learn to *move* in front of a camera.

WHOLESALE MODELING

The field of wholesale modeling is a wide, wonderful world all by itself. It's a world that is always in a state of excitement and change, and while the tempo quickens considerably with the two big seasonal showings, there is always something exciting to do and new people to meet. For every high-fashion photographic model in the limelight, there are hundreds of busy and successful wholesale, or showroom, models.

A girl needn't be a ravishing beauty to be a wholesale model, though it's surprising how many beauties there are. Nor does she have to have the slimness that is a prerequisite for most photographic modeling. Types and sizes are not as severely limited for the showrooms, and there is quite a bit more leeway in figures as well as facial qualities. A good figure within a certain size range and an attractive face are important, of course, but equally essential to a successful wholesale model is her ability to communicate the mood of a costume. And she must do it smoothly, effortlessly, and quickly. To a buyer, time is money. The model who can show off all the good points of a garment to her audience—which often may consist of only one person—as quickly and as graphically as possible is the model who will go far in the wholesale field.

The two major seasons in the fashion cycle are fall and spring. There are lesser showings throughout the year, but these are the two main events. To get the appropriate clothes into stores all over the country at the proper time, manufacturers must stay six months ahead of consumption. The manufacturers' season for the fall line comes up the preceding spring, while spring clothes are shown the previous fall.

Market Week

When people think of wholesale modeling, they invariably think of Market Week. There is a wide range of types and sizes needed for this, as the market is varied. A girl must be alert, enthusiastic, poised, and not afraid to work.

A warm personality is invaluable in this particular field. You must be able to work rapidly, without appearing rushed. You should know how to show your costume to advantage, with composure, and a great deal of feeling for your clothes. You will use your hand positions to play up the lines of the garment, without obviously using a great display of hands, to show details of the garment, the lining, or to change the scarf. You will show how a jacket is opened and removed.

Each manufacturer will have his own interpretation of the type of model he wants. It might be you.

Market Week is an important week. There is a great flurry of activity going on, and people are constantly under pressure. You should learn to arrive on time, with your planned schedule and your most perfectly groomed appearance. Don't ever be caught saying:

"I didn't have time for a manicure. My nails look terrible!"

"I forgot to bring an extra pair of stockings!"

"May I borrow your comb?"

"Does anybody have a pin?"

"I forgot to bring enough shoes," or "I forgot to clean my shoes!"

Just because you're not doing one big fashion show and your job is a regular one in the wholesale market, there's no need to become careless. So many of our girls tend to do this, but remember that the girl who makes it to the top is the one who always has that bandbox appearance.

Duties of a Wholesale Model

You must understand the different types of wholesale modeling. First, there is the girl who works for the manufacturer and is exactly the right size for the clothes made on the sample model. She will show the fashions to the buyers as they come in to give their orders.

Second, she may only work during Market Week. Extra girls are needed, but they still will have to be the size that the particular manufacturer shows. If she works in an apparel mart, she will work in one room, showing the buyer a different costume every time she comes out. There may be one model, or half a dozen.

Third, a girl may be a sample model. Sometimes the designer will drape clothes on a particular model whose looks are not important. It's the shape of her body that counts. She is used for the size and shape of her figure because those are the exact measurements the designer wants, and another girl will actually model the costume.

Fourth, she may be a sample and a wholesale model. In other words, the sample clothes are made and draped on her, literally made to her figure. Then she may model them afterward. Sometimes a girl is good enough to do both.

Let's assume that you have a job with a particular manufacturer. You're in a room and several buyers come in. The director or the designer will say, "Mary, go put on number 826," or "Let's show them numbers 128 and 345."

You go back into the dressing room, put on the number requested, come out smoothly and quickly, make a picture, and do a turn. The director has the number, and probably the designer will talk about it. You're helping to sell that costume, so the way you show it is important.

You may even feel free to point out a detail in the costume, perhaps the lining or something slightly hidden. This is your obligation to the designer.

Show the garment quickly, then go back and dress in the other costume. Come out again. You might state clearly and distinctly, "This is number 128. It's imported tweed from France and has a pure silk lining. It's $72.50."

This is repeated all day long—eight hours a day. Different buyers come in, but the routine is the same. It's a rather relaxed—though generally hurried—atmosphere. You may not always have the best conditions in which to dress. The showrooms are usually pleasant for the buyers, but they're limited in space, so that dressing-room comfort is sometimes sacrificed.

When you first apply for a job in wholesale modeling and the management asks you to try on a costume, model it to the best advantage. Never ask, "How do I model this?"

Step out with knowledge and confidence, and your viewer will know that you are aware of the way to show clothes.

Learn to listen and adjust to any instructions that may be given you. Every designer or manufacturer will want to show his garment in a certain way. You will have to be quick to adapt and use the modeling methods suggested to you, whether you agree or not. You may know a better way but, until you've been employed longer, it's strictly a matter of pleasing the employer. In time you may be able to ask if he'd like to see it this way or how would he feel about a slight change. Until then, though, it's best to do it the way you've been instructed.

I hope you'll have an opportunity to step out and use your initiative. Walk out then and model it *your* way. Your employer may be so pleased with the way you've done it that he'll find it's better than the suggestions he had in mind.

Press Showings

These are the very first showings of a designer's clothes before the public sees them. This is a very exciting time. The anticipation of a new season's showings is always heady and exhilarating. Model agencies will be called upon weeks in advance with requests for certain size models. The same size as the sample model, and probably six models will be needed. They will possibly be all different types in coloring, but they all must be the same size.

There is usually a rehearsal before the showing, so that the designer can see how the costumes will look on each model, and any necessary changes can be made rapidly and efficiently.

At press showings, the press and potential buyers in the audience will fill the room. The staging can range from a simple platform to an elaborate revolving stage, or it can be a carpet running down the center with the audience tiered—in as many rows as the room will allow—on either side. There is generally only a very small area for the models.

Remember, the press is in a hurry. They want to see as much as possible in as short a time as possible. A model may find herself assisting the other models. You may get the feeling that it's the opening night of a Broadway show because of all the rush and excitement. In a way, it *is* an opening. These clothes have not been seen by anyone except the designer and the people employed by the designer. It's all very hush-hush and top-secret and now—for the very first time— the collection will be viewed by potential buyers and the press.

Imagine that you're one of six models who have been selected. You've had your fittings. You've had a rehearsal. You know everything is just right for you. You're usually in very cramped quarters in the back, and the appropriate staging has been set up in front.

The showing must be fast and smooth and efficient. In some cases, you will have to speak. You probably also will carry the number of the costume modeled, so that the audience sees the number as well as hears it mentioned. You will be waiting in line, and every girl will have her position number and will keep that number throughout the show—1 through 6. When No. 1 has finished modeling, No. 2 will follow immediately. There is always a model showing; never a lull. This is most important. When it is time for you to step out there, do it.

All right. You step out into the spotlight—if there is a spotlight— and you're apt to be holding a number. You would say, "This is No. 1020; pure silk imported from Italy; lined in pure silk; $52.50." Or this would be said by a commentator or narrator.

You will walk quickly, do your turns at the proper places, turn again, and make your exit. The next model will follow you. Quickly make your changes and go on again. Often there is no commentator, and a girl will have to announce this herself. If there is a commentator, fine. You won't have to say anything. Just model quickly and smoothly, and always be waiting for your turn onstage.

In spite of the rushing, *do not be careless*. Be all business. Help others if you have time, and avoid chatter and extra talk backstage. Don't forget a belt, or a scarf, or gloves. Everything you're supposed to be showing should be remembered. This is important. Some models write accessories to model on a card for each costume. It's a safe check.

Remember, buyers are not an audience of leisurely women watching a fashion show. They are all business. Don't expect an avalanche of applause unless something truly outstanding should be created by the designer. The applause will be heard at the end of the showing.

A word of warning to the new model who is doing a show for a designer where the other girls have shown his or her clothes before. These models are old-timers. When you've been hired and find that the other models have been with the designer before, you must re-member you aren't in the "clique" yet. They have a little feeling of belonging once they have been called on twice or more. Don't try to push your way in. Be sociable and pleasant, and do a good job. Time will take care of your "belonging." Just be patient and smile. You are more or less on probation during your first show. You eventually will meet many interesting people in wholesale modeling. You'll make your own friends. Don't mar your chances for a proper place in it before you've even begun.

Concentrate on the following do's and don'ts:

ON THE "DO" SIDE

Do be dependable.
Do be neat, energetic.
Do be alert to business.
Do model well.
Do be charming. Your personality is important.

ON THE "DON'T" SIDE

Don't drink on the job.
Don't flirt.
Don't date a client. In unusual circumstances, you would discuss this with your employer.
Don't be temperamental.
Don't be too sensitive. You will work with artists and must learn to let slights—real or imagined—rub off a little.
Don't gossip. You may talk about people and things, but in a nice way. Models only hurt themselves by being destructive to anyone else.

There are some five thousand showroom models at work in New York alone, and more in Dallas, Los Angeles, San Francisco, and Chicago. And many more. The rate of pay is steady and you're on a weekly salary. The work is more relaxed in off seasons, of course, but otherwise you're under a lot of pressure. You will learn to take this in stride, because that's what makes for so much excitement in each new season's showings. It's a dependable job, and many girls give up the hectic work of doing single fashion shows for different clients, and enjoy working for one designer or manufacturer.

When showing a complete line, the manufacturer may have to hire extra models but usually one girl will work all year round. There may actually be two girls—the sample girl and the wholesale model—or a sample girl who does both. You should know how to write up orders and also be a salesgirl. You should help keep the office clean.

You're a little bit of everything. Always remember that there should be a relaxed atmosphere, whether you're showing for one buyer at a time or doing a full show.

You'll find that most showrooms have one model, or two at the most, with one modeling at a time. It's interesting to see how it's done in some of the apparel marts, though. In some of the larger showrooms, such as the Dallas Apparel Mart, there will be three to six models showing at one time.

I can't help but think how invaluable the experience of wholesale modeling can be. You learn the importance of color and fabric and line in buying and selling. Sometimes this experience serves as a definite stepping stone to an executive position in the fashion world. It can take you far beyond being a wholesale model, and this training should not be taken lightly.

RETAIL MODELING

The modeling of garments that are ready for sale is called Retail Modeling. This type of modeling is used in the fashion section or salon of a department store, or in a women's wear specialty shop.

The modeling is usually done by walking from one customer to another in the salon or throughout the store. The duties of the retail model are similar to those of the wholesale model. The rules are the same—the objective is to sell. However, in working with many different types of designers instead of just one, she will need to be more versatile. The garments to be modeled have already been selected by the store and they will carry the various designers' labels.

The retail model has to adapt herself and be able to change her appearance more often. She will have to be on her toes and be up to exacting demands with the aid of accessories, hairstyles, and makeup. Here is where hairpieces are useful. The model should be able to change her mood and style completely to fit those of the designer's clothes, but at the same time she must reflect a warm and distinctive personality which belongs to her alone.

The retail model is usually hired by the department store or the specialty shop. She is their employee and must please them. In addition to showing off their wares, she must be instrumental in selling them.

This mode of modeling is also used in the showing of the complete line of a designer's individual collection, known in the trade as a trunk showing, with orders ready to be taken.

A typical showing of a collection, or trunk showing, usually would be advertised in the local newspapers several days ahead of the event. The ad might read as follows:

Bonwit Teller is presenting
So-and-So's new Spring Collection.

Informal modeling 2 to 4 P.M., on the Sixth Floor
Monday through Friday ——————— (dates)

The Public Is Invited.

Larry Aldrich trunk showing at Fanny's in Las Vegas. Model Mark Griswold (left) has finished modeling in the salon and is ready to change into another style from the complete collection that is available for customers to see. A customer may request the model to wear a particular style for her to view. Orders are then taken for the customer's size, fabric, and color request.

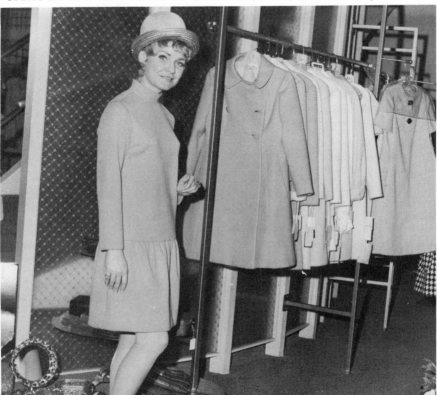

Salon Modeling

The salon is usually prepared in advance, with chairs lined up on either side of the runway or stage. The models come out one at a time, while the commentator gives a detailed description of the costume and its price. Several turns will be made so that everyone in the room will be able to see all angles of the costume. This is a very important part of modeling, as every customer in the room deserves a complete picture. This is a selling point, and the model is selling!

The model makes her exit smoothly, never giving the appearance of being rushed. The next model will follow immediately. However, a certain amount of rushing will be necessary when changing into the next costume so as to be ready for the next appearance.

In salon modeling—formal or informal—the model who is hired permanently is more relaxed. She knows the customers who constantly return to that shop. She is an ambassador of good will, and a salesgirl along with it.

Informal Modeling

Informal modeling may follow a fashion show or a trunk showing. This is modeling throughout a department store fashion section or a specialty shop during a specified period of time—usually one to two hours.

There normally will be more than one model, and a complete formal showing before the informal modeling.

The model shows the costumes one at a time, walking up to the customer and giving details of each garment, making sure to show all angles. If the featured designer has requested that orders be taken, that will be another duty to perform. (Usually saleswomen take the orders.)

Some department stores have adopted a rather fascinating practice in modeling, one that's most effective. The models stand and pose as mannequins in unexpected places in the fashion departments. It's quite a shock to see a girl suddenly walk away slowly and another girl take her place. This is especially startling to people who have just come off the elevator, and suddenly see a presumed mannequin come to life!

Happily for the weak-hearted, this isn't always the case. Most informal modeling is done by simply walking from one customer to another in the department.

For the convenience of the model and the customer, some department stores leave the price tag hanging from the garment. However, others do not practice this. It depends entirely on the management.

Do learn to know the customers' likes and dislikes.

Do work through your coordinator and keep the customer's interests at heart. Let her know you are interested in her fitting and color problems, if any.

Do model what your customer likes. She likes personal attention.

Don't chitchat with customers any longer than necessary to convey interest and warmth.

The best advice is to have warm, genuine concern for your customers' desires, and eagerness to please, and a knowledge of the merchandise so that you know what you're talking about.

Tearoom Modeling

Informal modeling branches out into tearoom modeling. The tearoom is an ideal setting for viewing fashions while having luncheon.

The model approaches the tables, taking a model's stance, or whatever pose that is appropriate for the garment being worn. The model will identify the shop or the section of the department store she's model-

Lovely Lenz model Yvonne Mongeon, High Fashion Sophisticate model in her thirties, is very much in demand. She is shown during a luncheon fashion show at the Showboat Hotel, Las Vegas. Note her grace and warmth. This is essential for tearoom modeling. Save your nonsmiling modeling for stage and salon work.

Photo by Frank Valeri

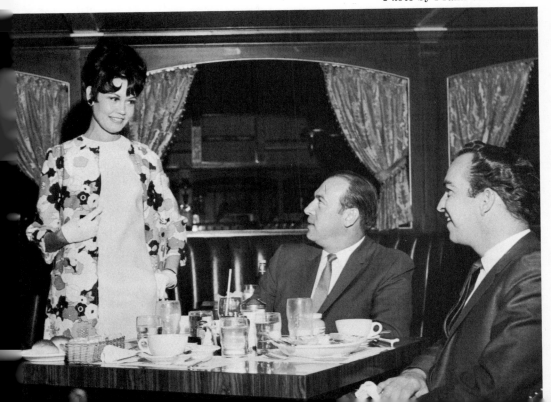

ing for, describe the garment, the fabric, the designer, and sometimes the price. Instructions regarding information to be given the customer vary; each store has a different method.

There are times when it is not necessary for the model to give pertinent facts. In these cases, the model answers only the questions asked directly by the patron. If interest is shown, give all the information requested.

The model will use a variety of turns in tearoom modeling. She will decide what will be the most effective ones to show the garments. Remember, these turns must be done gracefully and beautifully to show the garment to the best advantage, thus stimulating interest and possible sale.

If the director asks the models to stop at every table and do a turn, this must be done. Not one table should be passed up. Remember, you're out to sell clothes, and every area where you can be seen must be covered.

Tearoom modeling is generally done in the restaurant section of a department store or in a public restaurant. Some restaurants use a small stage, and in addition to using it, the models walk throughout the luncheon room.

In a department store, the models usually dress in the store's fashion section and go over to model in the tearoom, if it is nearby. Or they take the clothes from the fashion section to dressing rooms adjacent to the modeling area.

When a fashion show is presented at a restaurant the clothes will have to be transported to it where a small dressing room will be set up. All that is needed is a chair for each model, a clothes rack, and a mirror. A table would be a useful accessory, but it is not necessary.

Modeling clothes in a good restaurant where there is much activity and a large luncheon crowd can stimulate business, and this type of exposure is being used all over the country. I introduced this type of modeling in Las Vegas at the El Cortez Hotel, which has a dining room with a small stage, an ideal setting. The commentator stands at one side of the stage, and after the models have shown the clothes onstage, they step down into the dining room and stop at each table or booth to give the patrons a closer view of the costumes. Background music is provided.

Usually there is no runway or stage in a restaurant. A step-up platform or a one-step box to slightly elevate the girls is very helpful, but the restaurant owner may not want to invest in this extra prop. Therefore, the models would simply walk around the room, showing the clothes.

Whatever the setup—from a runway, to a stage, to a little box to step on, to a very short area consisting of two steps and maybe a

4-foot or 8-foot runway—the model must be conditioned for any setting. A good exercise would be for the model to try to visualize the various ways in which a restaurant could be set up, and so be ready for anything.

So much for the setting itself. Now, let's think of the model. Her responsibility, of course, is to sell the clothes she is modeling. She will, therefore, have to have complete information about the garments.

Remember, in our big productions and in regular fashion shows, the model is not required to talk, just to look beautiful. She is seen, but never heard. In tearoom modeling where the model is in close contact with the audience, her voice is going to help her tremendously. She must be aware of the sound of her voice and learn to speak with gaiety and enthusiasm.

She also must have a complete knowledge of fashion and be able to answer all questions regarding the garment so that she can give a complete description.

1. Know the color—when working with a new color, rather than just red, it may be cinnamon red, apple red, or tomato.

2. Know the type of garment—a dress, pantsuit, or whatever it happens to be.

3. Know the design. Is the costume A-line, a tunic, slim?

4. Know the fabric.

5. Know the details that should be mentioned—silk piping, lining, bound buttonholes, extremely unusual buttons, and so on. Any detail worth mentioning should be talked about.

6. Know the designer. This isn't always mentioned, but it should be known.

7. Know the price. It may not be asked, but it's a good idea to know it.

All of this may sound like a very tall order at first, but it's surprising how easily the information can be learned, especially after a model becomes very much aware of fashion.

At first, it might be well to write the information on a card, with possibly a duplicate for the commentator. Some commentators require this. The card will look like this:

> "I am wearing a red wool knit 3-piece suit, with long jacket and slim skirt. The detail is bone buttons in matching color. The designer is Sebastian, and the price is $125.00."

It might be well to practice by describing the garment you are wearing right now.

On a 4 by 6 card, print your name in the top left-hand corner and the shop's name in the top right-hand corner. Follow the example above, only this time, describe your own costume. Skip a line and describe your second costume in the same way, and so on. Remember the proper order: 1. color, 2. type of garment, 3. design, 4. fabric, 5. detail, 6. designer, 7. price.

The average tearoom model will show four to six changes. Four is an average. Approximately fifteen minutes are necessary to walk around a tearoom seating two hundred people. The average luncheon time for each customer is about one hour. If the model is working a two-hour luncheon, she may repeat the four garments. If the model has six costumes, two probably will be repeated. Since the average luncheon customer would not have been there for two hours, repeating would not present a problem as, likely, there would be a change of customers.

Should there be a fashion commentator, the model will make out the card listing the four (or six) changes. Use one card only, unless the commentator specifically requests a card for each costume. Either way, it's a most effective way of saving time. Sometimes it will not be necessary for the model to do this, especially if the commentator works in the store, knows the merchandise well, and has made quick notes herself on a sheet of paper.

Generally, however, my suggestion to a commentator would be for her to ask the models to fill in a card similar to the one the models write out. It will save her a great deal of time and make her task easier, and will be good training for the model. Once the model has the information, written down, she will remember what she's modeling for the customer, so the cards actually work well for the model and the commentator.

For instance, if there are six models with four cards each, it could be too much to handle. Twenty-four cards can be mixed up with unbelievable ease! On the other hand, if each card has four changes, there are only six cards to cope with. Each card has a number on it from 1 to 4, to correspond with the model as she comes out.

A tearoom model is apt to be on much more intimate terms with the audience, though this will vary.

IN DEPARTMENT STORES

Some department stores don't allow the model to talk; others do. We have found from personal experience that we get better sales results when the model talks. However, when there's a large area to cover, she won't have time to say much. This should be left to the management. It depends on what atmosphere is required.

In tearoom modeling, walk to the table, pause, and give a brief description of your garment, particularly details that the customer may not be aware of. Mention the fabric, the comfortable design of the suit, the designer, and the price if the store approves. Very often the price is not mentioned unless the customer asks for it.

You're at the table and now have—I hope—your customer's attention. You might say something like:

"Good afternoon. I'm modeling fashions from Alexander's sportswear department. This is a smart red wool imported Italian knit suit. The bone button detail is especially interesting for this new season's collection."

Smile, and turn. You may use a Model's Pivot, Three-Quarter French Turn, or Half Turn.

This brings us to an interesting point. A model who works tearooms must be sensitive to the customer. Some customers come to a tearoom for luncheon because they are definitely interested in fashions. Others come for luncheon and are not interested in fashions. You will soon learn to detect who is interested. If the customer is truly interested, then you give details. If you sense no interest, be brief, but courteous.

If you do see a spark of interest, you'll want to be more informative. If, for instance, you know the costume comes in a color that would be more attractive on her, you might tell her so. You might even say, "This garment comes in a beautiful shade of blue that would look well on you." Remember, you're trying to sell this garment.

IN RESTAURANTS

There's another phase of tearoom modeling that is becoming more popular—modeling in a restaurant. The model may or may not be required to transport the clothes she is to model. When she is requested to do this, there are a few things to remember. The model is responsible for the clothes. They must be returned in as good condition as when taken from the store. They should be carried in a plastic or cloth bag that has a bottom. If the garment should fall from the hanger, it will fall inside the bag and avoid becoming soiled. For extra protection, caution should be taken to secure the garment to the hanger so that it can't fall off.

Carry the clothes into the part of the restaurant which has been assigned as a dressing room. The girls will usually help each other dress, do the show, have lunch quickly (thirty minutes)—most restaurants donate the lunch—and take the clothes back to the shop.

As the model is responsible for the clothes until they are returned to the store, be certain that someone is with the clothes throughout the fashion show. If there is no assistant to do this, wait for a model to return before leaving the dressing room.

MAKE A REPORT

Always give a report on your assignment. We're assuming it's a *good* report, but always give a report of what happened at the luncheon to your fashion coordinator or the shop owner. That is the only way they will know how the clothes were accepted. Keep your eyes open, be alert, and be aware that you are representing the store and trying to sell its clothes. That's the reason you have the job, so be a good tearoom model.

Even in small cities, any particular place that has a luncheon crowd is an ideal place for a store to stimulate business. Even the few men scattered among the women are potential buyers.

Frequently, a fashion showing will include fashions from different shops. True, stores are in competition, but they all buy differently and their showings need not conflict. Each store benefits individually, and the customer is presented with a varied and interesting fashion show. In this type of showing, a coordinator is necessary and she will invite a number of shops to participate. This stimulates business for all and makes for a beautiful showing.

We have tearoom modeling at many places. Some shops use three or more models. They can afford individual shows and like to keep them exclusively theirs.

BASIC TECHNIQUES

Basically, you will use model's pivots. You may reach around and do a slow Three-Quarter French Turn, do Pivot Fours between tables: always use your hands correctly, and when you turn around, don't talk with your back to the table. Face your customers when talking. Finish your conversation directly to them.

The same rule applies in modeling jackets or coats. Open them up toward the table, then adjust them straight to show the back neatly as you turn. This is a weak area, I find.

You must learn to adjust garments on your body and present them beautifully to the front of the table. Straighten the jacket and, as you turn, the customer sees the back. The exception will be when you drop a coat or a jacket to reveal any unusual back interest of the dress. When you turn around, open a jacket or coat so that the inside can be seen.

DON'T BE A BORE!

In tearoom showing, a model must be sure she doesn't sound like a parrot! The fact that you are repeating the same facts at fifty or more tables makes it imperative for you to learn to vary the conversation.

For instance, you may mention the shop first at one time, the fabric second, and the detail third. Then switch it. Mention the shop in the middle of your sentence, if you like, but do change the wording so that you constantly don't repeat.

Occasionally you hear a model say:

"Good afternoon. I'm modeling fashions from the Vogue Salon. This is a 100-percent wool sport suit, and it is priced at $100.00."

Then she goes to the next table and says exactly the same thing. The next table, the same, and again and again. She soon sounds like a broken record. This is an example of what *not* to do.

You must be brief and to the point, and play it from different angles so that you don't end up sounding monotonous.

Review: Practice tearoom modeling. This would be most helpful in gaining experience. Ask a friend to sit at a table. Walk up to her and go through the routine you've just learned. Give the details, make the turns, smile, and go off to another table.

CONVENTION AND EXHIBIT MODELING

In convention and exhibit modeling, a girl is hired to promote a product. She is on exhibition, and actually is on exhibit herself. Sometimes she is called an exhibit or convention model as well as a promotional model.

Sparkling exhibit model Judi Moreo was selected during the "World Congress of Flight" convention (1968). Her job was to model a "Fashion for Flight" costume that consisted of eight different pieces, which she continually took off and on. Try doing this with fresh excitement five to eight hours a day! Another model explained computers all day long. Exhibit modeling is always varied.

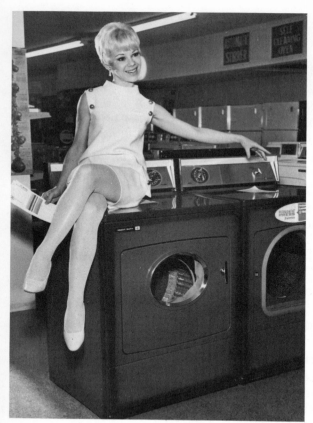

Pert Lenz model Wendy Rogers has been selected many times as an exhibit model. Here her assignment was to sit prettily on the washing appliance while she demonstrated it and handed out brochures to customers. Wendy is 5 feet tall, wears sizes 3 and 5.

Conventions are big business and models are very much in demand. When a convention is held in a large city, a model agency is called for attractive models who can assist in promoting particular products, and perform various duties. They may be attractive hostesses, standing or sitting beside the product, distributing brochures, or demonstrating the product to prospective buyers.

A pretty, appealing girl has proved to be an invaluable aid to sales. With an attractive girl showing the item, it sells better. It's that simple! The best investment convention promoters can make — and they know it — is to hire girls with charm and personality to show their products.

Convention modeling is one of the best branches of the profession. The rate of pay is good, and convention business is growing fast in every large city, as well as in many smaller ones.

Las Vegas, the convention capital of the West, hosted 235 trade shows in 1967. The figure has been rapidly rising every year. The city's ability to handle this large number of conventions has resulted from the fantastic development of convention and banquet facilities in the resort hotels along the famed Strip and in the nearby $9.5-million Convention Center.

The growing popularity of Las Vegas as the ideal convention city has been aided by the same factors that draw 14.5 million visitors to the city each year: gaming, perpetual sunshine, more than 25,000 first-class rooms, and almost unlimited entertainment and recreation.

Plans are now being considered to construct another 300,000-square-foot addition to the 90,000 feet of exhibit space that already covers five acres. This will allow a convention of any size in the world to visit Las Vegas.

These conventions need service in many ways, and one important area is hiring attractive models. So if your city has conventions, find out which model agency gives service to them.

You must look every inch a model and have that outgoing personality we have discussed in the previous chapters.

Rates of pay vary widely from city to city; indeed, from company to company. In Las Vegas, a convention model usually will be paid $40 to $50 a day, with a $25 minimum call. Five dollars an hour—or a $25 minimum call—is pretty average, but in some cities rates may go as low as a $15 minimum. In New York, I've seen models get from $100 to $250 a day. Obviously, the top rates go to the top models. Your pay will depend on your ability, the area in which you live, and the type of assignment that is requested. Extra talent demands a higher rate of pay.

We have many calls for models here in Las Vegas, and we place many of our girls in convention work. Not only do prospective employers want a model to be attractive—not necessarily beautiful, but attractive—but they insist on personality. She must have a warm, magnetic quality that will attract people and keep them interested in the product being displayed.

What will you have to know as a convention model? This is where finishing-school training is important. You should know how to sit properly, how to walk properly, and how to stand up beautifully on a platform. You should really know your basic modeling techniques, and this, again, is why this book should be so valuable to you.

How do you use your hands gracefully? How do you pick up an item to show its best points—and yours? How do you run your hand along the curve of an appliance to show the lovely lines of it? Each of these things is important, and if you learn modeling and how to be graceful, it will all come much more easily for you.

Your duties, primarily, are to understand the product. Ask for brochures that will help you familiarize yourself with it. Realize that your responsibility is to get people interested in the product, but once you have that interest, you must know what you're talking about. Naturally, you don't have to know all the inner workings of an item or a machine, but at least know the salient features. Don't be afraid to ask your employer questions about his product before you go out and answer questions people will ask you.

Be animated. You have to attract people to you. Don't just stand there and smile — or not smile — like a dummy. Do what your employer tells you. Exert yourself. Greet people. Everyone is a friend. If you can actually feel that everyone who passes your product is a friend to whom you're eager to tell all about it, your task will be much simpler. Put your heart into it. You'll get people interested and they'll be happy with you and, hopefully, with the product that you're promoting.

You can make a successful career of convention modeling alone, or you can fit it into other facets of the field. If you do work in the other branches of modeling, doing some convention work can be just what you need to keep you in the field on a full-time basis. In smaller cities, where photographic and television assignments are relatively scarce, convention modeling could be the answer.

TELEVISION MODELING

Modeling for television breaks down roughly into two categories — making commercials and modeling fashions on certain specialized shows. Types of models differ for commercials and TV-fashion modeling. Commercials, of course, offer far more leeway.

Modeling for Commercials

Casting directors want the regular, average-looking person for commercials. This is so that the viewer will be able to identify with the model and the product. The commercial model, in many cases then, is the average housewife. Often she isn't even average-looking! Producers go so far in trying to be realistic that sometimes their subjects aren't even believable.

Besides the "average" trademark, producers look for unusual types who can hold your interest or, possibly, cause you to smile. With so many of today's commercials leaning toward the frankly funny, a model who can put over a rueful sort of humor will be very much in demand. A gamine quality is good. Sometimes a commercial will require a model who is actually overweight, or homely, or shrill-voiced.

Naturally we don't want any of you to be any of these things deliberately, but if you should be a little heavy or not the most beautiful girl in the world, at least you know that there may be a place in modeling for you.

You will find the average-looking person is used in commercials which sell detergents, household items and appliances, headache and cold remedies, deodorants, and that sort of thing. For shampoos, beauty soaps and cosmetics, travel, or cigarettes, you have to be a glamour girl. There are a few occasional exceptions, but generally there is no compromise there. If you're modeling fashions for television, you must photograph well and you must be very slim. TV adds extra poundage, so you'll simply have to weigh less to qualify.

Possibly the most attractive thing in modeling for commercials is that attractive word "residuals." Even the layman knows what that is. It's the extra pay — on a sliding scale — that you get every time your commercial is shown!

Your basic pay can be as low as $61.50, depending on whether you have lines, or do a walk-on, or just a voice-over. (Voice-overs — speaking parts that are heard while other people are actually on camera — are usually done by actors. If you have a beautiful speaking voice, though, you might look into this.) What boosts your pay into what are sometimes astronomical figures are the residuals. These payments are based on the number of times your commercial is rerun within each thirteen-week cycle and in what particular metropolitan areas it is shown. Should your commercial be shown often enough over enough stations during a long period of time, your earnings can go up into the thousands for just one commercial!

Two unions in the United States have been instrumental in raising these income possibilities for models. They are the Screen Actors Guild (SAG) and the American Federation of Television and Radio Artists (AFTRA). SAG operates in the area of films; AFTRA concerns television that is live or videotaped. SAG and AFTRA have agreements with many leading TV stations throughout the country and with all the leading networks, but not all cities have union agreements that cover modeling for television.

If you want to appear on TV programs that have agreements with AFTRA or SAG, you'll have to join these unions. You have to join AFTRA *before* your first appearance, but SAG will allow you to appear in one TV film without joining. After thirty days, however, you may not appear in any other TV films without joining SAG. Initiation fee for each organization is $200, but if you already belong to one you can join the other at half-rate. Your future dues are based on your TV earnings.

As you can see, modeling for television commercials can be very lucrative, and the field is wide open as far as types and appearance are concerned. You have more opportunity here, but you also have to be more versatile. You'll have to be able to act, for one thing. You won't be aiming for the Academy Award or the Emmy, but you must be able to do simple, believable acting. You might even be called upon to sing a little or do a dance step or two. You must be able to change your looks pretty radically—makeup, hairpieces, and a knowledge of clothes are your allies here—so you won't be easily identified with any one product. Being identified with a single product can be great for a while and pile up the residuals, but it can play hob with your availability for other work. You're typed. This, of course, is up to you. Maybe you'd rather be rich!

Fashion Modeling

Now that roughly more than 10 percent of the nation has color television, and more and more color sets will be installed in homes, more fashion modeling will be shown on TV. Some of it will be live, but much of it will be taped.

This is an area that requires a slightly different technique from that used in salon or fashion-show modeling. Your pattern of pivots and turns will depend largely on the amount of space you have to work in.

If you have to stay in a small studio, where you have to remain practically in place and can't walk around much, you will do things a little bit differently. You may have a small runway or a bigger studio. You may even occasionally be in an outside area where the cameras have been brought in. In this case, you can model on the runway as you always do.

The basic rule in television modeling is to model a little bit slower. Don't be quick with your hands. Be very smooth and fluid. You can use all of your steps if you have the space to do so. But if you're going to model right in front of the camera, here are some points to observe.

Open with an attractive pose and give the audience—and the commentator—time enough to adjust to looking at the costume, then change your hand positions as you turn slowly to show the back, remembering to look over your shoulder and see if you're still with the audience as you come around. Change your hand position again, possibly stepping to the side to change it. Step back. It all depends on how much time you've been allotted in front of the camera. You may have fifteen seconds, thirty seconds, maybe more, to show one garment.

TV time is expensive and you probably won't be allowed to show too much detail.

Except for lavish productions on some of the late-night shows like Johnny Carson's, where models will arrive dripping with priceless furs and jewels—and be guarded by Brinks or Burns—there isn't much fashion modeling done in prime-time TV. You'll see more of it on morning programming. Try to look at some of the morning TV and catch the fashion modeling.

You'll see that hands are used a bit more, I should say considerably more, above the waist. To show a ruffle or neckline, the TV model will bring her hand up higher than she would if she were modeling onstage. She apparently wants to emphasize the commentator's words with this hand gesture. I would prefer to get her away from this position and do something else.

I'm partial to keeping the hands away from the face or chest area, unless the model is actually moving something. You don't want to look as if you're pointing to things. Yet, we often see models doing just that, probably because they're being directed to do so.

Timing is so important here that I think you ought to work on it. I would suggest you take a stop watch or a clock with a sweep-second hand, and stand in front of a mirror. Now time yourself for a fifteen-second showing of a garment. Just make a turn, change your hand positions twice, and your fifteen seconds are about gone. If you do this and step to the side, you might just possibly make one more change of a foot position. Practice this with a thirty-second showing, and then a forty-five. You'll probably not get much more time.

TV fashion shows are fun and exciting but, like any showing, must be handled according to the wishes of your coordinator. You may not have a coordinator, but only a director. Most morning shows are relaxed and informal; some shows that are filmed for a special collection or department store are more formal, and the late-night fashion segments are often frankly hilarious. On one of these, it's perfectly all right to laugh. In fact, with some of the zany goings-on and the host's comments, you won't be able to help it!

The following pictures were taken at a recent fashion show at the Tropicana Hotel in Las Vegas. Each model had to pose very quickly for the photographer. Note the positions of the legs, feet, body, head, eyes, arms, and hands. You can learn to pose just as quickly and effectively by practicing the suggestions in the chapter on fashion photography.

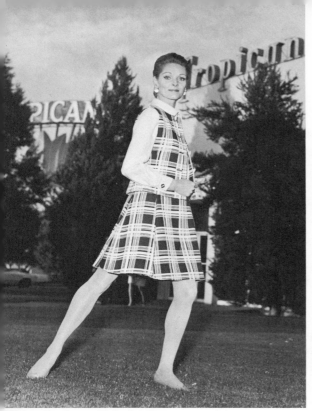

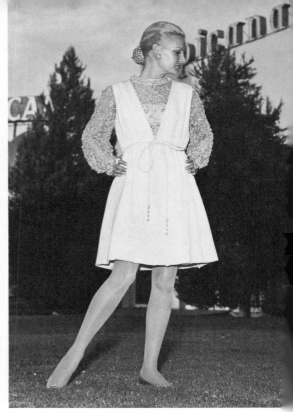

Designer Malcolm Starr

Designer Malcolm Starr

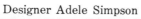
Designer Adele Simpson

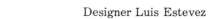
Designer Luis Estevez

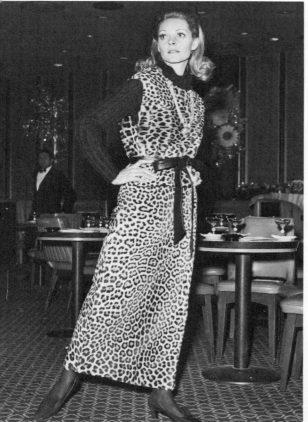

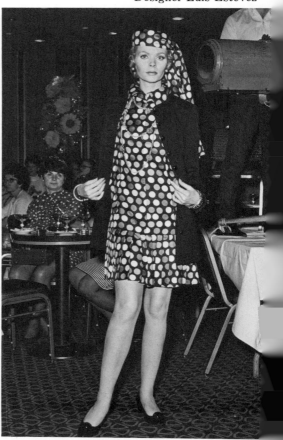

9

PREPARING YOURSELF FOR ASSIGNMENTS

Beauty Care and Wardrobe

By now you've learned your basic techniques of modeling, how to work a stage or a runway, handle groups and finales, and how to model accessories. You know what types of assignments are available and how to do them.

Now it's time to learn how to make the most of *yourself*, personally. This chapter is all about taking care of the outer you so that you'll appear at your absolute best at all times and in all places.

This chapter covers makeup, grooming, hair care and hairpieces, your figure, wardrobe and fittings, and, most important, a special section I like to call my "Model's Bag of Tricks." This includes a group of hints, tips, and techniques that help to save the day when something unexpected comes up in the line of duty.

YOUR MAKEUP

A person hurrying past on Manhattan's busy West 55th Street might miss seeing a modest little plate-glass window and an unobtrusive doorway at No. 150. The window houses as compact a collection of cosmetics as you'll see anywhere, and through that doorway pass some of the most beautiful women in the world. This is the Make-Up Center, the boutique of Dick and Carlo La Torre, makeup experts extraordinaire.

The La Torres are makeup consultants to most of the top models in the business, as well as advisors to the many young hopefuls

141

just starting out. In the past few years, the brothers have evolved complete new fashions in cosmetics and launched entirely new concepts in makeup techniques. They created their own line of specially formulated makeup with the professional model in mind. It is called, appropriately enough, "Onstage." We use it in our school.

Dick and Carlo are often called in to handle specific problems for some of our greatest beauties, though, naturally, their lips are sealed as to the who's and the how's. In the necessary absence of detail, it should be a comforting thought to beginners to know that even some of the top professional beauties have flaws that need to be minimized and problems that need to be solved.

The La Torres give workshops at the Models' Association of America conventions. They are personal friends of mine, and Dick has held workshops at our school. I thought you might like to hear some of their views on makeup, so I asked them for some tips and pointers especially for this book. Dick was the spokesman, as Carlo was kept busy tending to business as usual!

Basically, according to Dick, there is a subtle difference between everyday makeup and a model's makeup. Bright lights tend to wash out color, so a model's makeup must be just a touch more definite, more dramatic. Not garish, but more defined.

When you're going on an assignment—unless it's for a cosmetic company—have your makeup completely on. Time is money, and the person who is hiring you—photographer, coordinator, designer, or whoever—is paying you from the moment you walk in to the moment you walk out. If you spend half an hour or more of that expensive time putting on your makeup, chances are that you won't be hired a second time.

Dick isn't giving any specific makeup tricks for you to follow. He says—and I agree—that each face is different, and flaws and problems are highly individualized. He does, however, give us a few general tips that should help basically. After you learn them, you can apply them to your own needs. You'll have to practice and experiment, until you hit on the combination that's right for you.

Contouring in Specific Areas

Contouring is simply the art of sculpting the features with lights and darks. Dark colors cause planes to recede; light ones make them prominent. If you want to make a feature appear smaller—a nose or chin, for instance—use your dark contouring makeup. Want to play up a feature? Use your light makeup. That's really all there is to it. It's up to you to learn what you should highlight and what you should play down.

HIGHER CHEEKBONES.   High cheekbones have always been considered desirable in a model's face. To achieve this effect, lightly brush on a soft brown shadow in the pocket of the cheek. Suck in the cheek area, and just under the bone and in the pocket a darker shading will give the effect of lifting the cheekbone higher. A touch of iridescent overbase at the highest ridge of the cheekbone will highlight the bone structure even more.

LARGER NOSE. Use a white toner under foundation and a lighter foundation on the nose. Blend carefully.

THINNER NOSE. Brush soft brown powdered shading down the sides of the nose and around the nostrils. Blend the edges with fingers, and this will miraculously create a thinner nose.

SHORTER NOSE. Brush soft brown shading around the tip of the nose, and a transformation seemingly takes place. Add white down the top of the nose.

REDUCE SIZE OF CHIN. You may either use a darker shade of foundation or brush on the darker shading around the edge of the chin, blending it carefully over the curve. See how your chin recedes?

HIDE EXTRA FLESH UNDER CHIN.   A small shadow of dark shading brushed on in a triangle under the chin does wonders to remove that fleshy look.

ENLARGE CHIN AREA. Apply white toner on the chin before applying foundation. Blend a lighter shade of foundation over the chin. Here, again, you may add a touch of iridescent overbase to further bring out the chin.

NARROW A WIDE AREA BETWEEN EYES. Brush on soft brown shadow with a fluff brush to shade the sides of the nose near the corners of the eyes and blend shading down the nose. Blend it over the top center part of the eye structure. This will create a better bone structure from the eye and down the sides of the nose.

CAMOUFLAGE PUFFINESS AROUND EYES. To cause puffy shadows around the eyes to recede, brush the brown shading lightly over the areas. If you need more color, blend a light touch of dry brush-on rouge on top of the brown contouring and blend it all with a fluff of transparent powder.

There is a special brush for each area of contouring. This is most important for a perfect job.

As you work with shadowing, think of yourself as a photographer moving lights around you to create shadow and highlights where you need them. Pick up a fashion magazine and analyze the dark and the light planes of each model's face. When you see those interesting shadows, they may be due partly to the photographer's lights and partly to the model's skill with makeup.

Shading will vary in intensity. This will depend on the type of model assignment you're making up for, and the effect that is desired. Every model uses contouring somewhere—to perfect her bone structure or to emphasize it.

Blemishes

"You shouldn't have any." Dick is very definite about this. He maintains that if you get enough sleep, eat the proper foods, and are scrupulous about keeping your skin clean, you just won't have any blemishes. An occasional blemish can usually be camouflaged by covering with "TV Touch" before applying foundation. Nevertheless, if you have excessively oily skin and clogged pores at this stage of the game, you need help! Try this treatment for two weeks or longer and see the difference. Be very dogmatic about daily routine.

Wash your face morning and late afternoon for one minute with any good soap that agrees with your skin. Use a clean washcloth every time. Rinse extremely well—until squeaky clean. Apply antiseptic on any blemish before applying makeup. Once a day spend fifteen minutes in cleaning, steaming, removing ripe blemishes. This is usually best accomplished before bedtime. This is the order in which it should be done:

A. Cream neck and face well with a water soluble cleansing cream. Wash off well with washcloth and water. This helps soften the hard surface of the clogged pore.

B. While the face is wet, rub Beauty Scrub over entire face and work into skin gently for two minutes. Spend extra time on problem areas. The grains help remove flakiness and help scrub out surface-clogged pores. Rinse off very well.

C. Steam your face. This can be accomplished with the facial sauna that is on the market now, or do it yourself the barbershop way. Take a face towel and, while holding the dry ends, run very hot water in the center of the towel. Twist the water out of the towel and place against the face; fold over the dry ends to hold in the steam. Repeat this three times. Then check your skin carefully for blemishes that look ready to remove. The removing of blackheads should be done with great care.

D. Removing blackheads should be done with an instrument you can buy at most drugstores. It is called a blackhead remover, and is a small steel instrument with two holes, one at either end. You place either hole over the clogged pore and press gently. If the blackhead does not come out easily, wait until another time. You do not want to bruise the skin. It is also important to let none of the clogged pore matter touch the surface of your skin. Rinse the instrument off with steaming hot water or alcohol and continue your job of removing any more blackheads. Rinse your face with cold water and apply antiseptic to every blemish.

Be very diligent about this daily skin care. Never, never go to bed without cleaning your skin well.

Again, see that you have sufficient sleep. Schedule yourself so that you are not rushed. Hurry and worry are not helpful to an oily skin condition. Avoid chocolate and fatty foods as they aggravate your skin problem. See that you have all the essential foods per day. Three meals a day, even if they are light meals. Take a vitamin food supplement if you are a poor eater. Be realistic about your problem and what is necessary to help yourself.

False Eyelashes

There is nothing that enhances the model's eyes more than long, thick eyelashes. There are dozens of styles and designs, from the little half-lashes to be worn at the outer corners to the double- and triple-fringed lashes that can be attached underneath your own. The shape and size of your eyes—as well as the prospective occasion—will determine which type you choose. Always use a good surgical adhesive every time you apply your lashes. This is how you apply false eyelashes:

A. Sit down and tilt a magnifying mirror to the point where you are looking down into the mirror.

B. Take a toothpick and apply a white rim of surgical glue along the entire edge of the false lash.

C. Take the lash and hold the center part at the tip edge with tweezers. Check to see you are holding the lash correctly. You want the shorter edge near the nose; also lashes curl up, not down. This may sound silly, but it is easy to do things backwards in a mirror. Looking down into your mirror, place the center edge of the false lash at the center part of your own top lash root. Release the tweezers and pick up one end of the false lash at the tip end again and pull it down into place against the root base of your own lash. Release again and pick up the other end of the lash and place it against the root base of your own lash. Take an orange stick and gently press along the edges to be certain all the base is touching. With some practice, you will be applying your false lashes in less than a minute. Some girls like to start at one edge and work to the other end of the lash. Try both ways and see which is easier for you. Because the eye curves out to the center part more than to the edges, it is easier for most girls to apply lashes there first, but like so many tricks in makeup, results that are fast and easy for you are what you strive for.

INDIVIDUAL LASHES

It may be necessary for you to be able to add individual lashes for various effects. This is accomplished very easily. You may buy an inexpensive pair of fine black lashes, or buy a long strip that can be cut into either a full lash or into strips of varying lengths. If you want an individual lash (one hair), merely pull it away from the strip it's attached to. Pick it up with tweezers and dip the end into a spot of glue, or you can touch it to the tip of the tube. Place the lash on top of your own in the same manner as we explained with the strip, only this time you will be doing one at a time. I personally like cutting about two or three hairs off the strip of lash and applying little clusters at the edge of your own lash. This looks lovely on the outer edge of your own top lashes, or add a second layer on top of a false pair you have on.

BOTTOM LASHES

Whether you add one lash or a small cluster of lashes to the bottom of your own lashes, it is done in the same manner, just as we've instructed for the top lash application. The only difference is that you must remember to turn the lash so it will curl *down*, and place the lash under your bottom lash, not on top. If any trimming is needed, take a pair of blunt scissors and cut the length off at an angle after the lashes are on. Keep the outer edge of the bottom lash longer. You may want to add lashes on the outer half of your own lash or make a complete line across. Look at the current fashion trends in the fashion magazines and study the models' eye makeup very carefully. At the moment, it is the fluffy-lash look that is in vogue.

Eyebrows

They can enhance—or ruin—your entire expression. For eyebrows, we have specific instructions, and we'll go into them a few pages farther on.

Here is the basic beauty program we suggest. We use Onstage

makeup throughout because it's so specifically geared to a model's needs, but you can use any pure makeup that corresponds with what we are suggesting.

Fourteen Steps in a Perfect Makeup

1. CLEANSE. Your skin must be absolutely clean before a dab of makeup goes on. Use a water-soluble cleansing cream.

2. FRESHEN. A freshener removes soil and refines pores. Use cotton for applying. Excellent to use before a quick touch-up of makeup.

3. MOISTURIZE. Apply moisturizer after cleansing and always before makeup. Use an enriched moisturizer for dry skin, a regular for normal or oily skin. It is well to remember that it's not an oil you're applying. The object is to replace moisture in the skin. When you apply moisture cream, it plumps up the skin in very much the same manner a prune smooths out when soaked in water. Your makeup will go on more smoothly and your skin will appear more youthful. Use a small amount, and don't forget your neck.

4. TV TOUCH (or white toner). This is the magic lightener you will use around the eyes and over areas you want brought out or covered up if they are dark in appearance. Blend it around the eyes and over every dark spot before applying foundation. Use it sparingly and blend out the edges. There is a special cream type and there is also a liquid. For the very young skins, the cream type is best. For more mature skin, use the liquid white toner.

5. APPLY FOUNDATION. You want your skin to have a creamy appearance. There are various foundation consistencies. If you have a perfect skin, a liquid will be your choice in most cases. If you need more coverage, use a firmer creamy foundation and apply with the fingertips or a damp sponge. Always blend with a tissue around the hairline and the edges under the chin and neck, blending into a V-shape under the chin. You shouldn't be able to see where it ends, and you don't want to carry it too low on the neck as the makeup will soil your clothing. A beautiful foundation is the basis of a lovely makeup. Select a color close to your own skin or a shade darker.

6. APPLY ROUGE. A slight blush of color on the cheekbone will brighten the eyes and give you a healthy look. The blush you see on a baby's face is what you want. There are cream rouges, dry rouges,

liquid rouges. I prefer an iridescent liquid rouge to blend on after applying foundation. Apply a dot under the eyes on top of your cheekbones. Blend it on top of the bone structure and just under where a hollow should be. Stay about half an inch away from the nose for a normal bone structure. Do not go below the nose area. It should be a blended triangle to the hairline, or stop just short of the hairline if your face is very narrow.

A blush color will look good on anyone, but you can lean to the golden tones if you desire this in your makeup coloring. If you use the dry brush-on rouge, apply it after you have set your foundation with translucent powder. Use it in the same area as given above, and simply brush it on.

7. APPLY POWDER. This sets your makeup and it will last longer under hot lights. (Look for a new product that you can spray on the face to set the makeup for extremely hot lights.) Take a powder brush and dip both sides into the powder. Blot the powder over the entire face, starting at the neckline. Then brush excess off lightly. Always brush down fine hairs at the end of your brushing.

8. EYEBROWS. You do them at this stage, but since it's such a long technique we have a separate section on them below.

9. CONTOURING. This will start with the eye shadow you select to brush on. It may be the white our model has selected (we call it toast), or you may use brown or another color. You may want to experiment with three colors to see what effect each one gives to your eyes. After the shadow is brushed on, you will start contouring the bone structure areas that need help. Refer back to the contouring section and see what your face needs. Then follow the instructions that are appropriate. Using the theory of darks and lights, work to your individual needs.

10. APPLY EYELINER. A smooth, thin eyeliner may take hours of practice, but it must be perfect. Mix your own brown and gray combination if you find the color from the container isn't perfect for you. Many models blend their own color combinations. Check the liner color against your hair, brow, and eye coloring. Looking down into an up-tilted magnifying mirror is the best way to achieve easy results. Brace your little finger against the cheekbone and draw the line at the base of your own lash. It's usually best to start near the nose area. Be certain there is a fine point at both ends. Use a cotton Q-Tip to perfect a line or correct a mistake. Copy our model's look.

11. APPLY MASCARA. Mascara will make your lashes look longer and thicker. In most cases, black is used. Put it onto the top as well as under upper lashes for a thicker appearance. Bottom lashes should be done also. Check to separate them, if needed. I might add that some models do not use mascara except on the bottom lashes. They feel that false lashes on the top are sufficient. Experiment both ways to find out which is best for you.

12. APPLY FALSH LASHES. This is when you apply your false lashes. Refer back to the section that gives instructions in detail.

13. APPLY LIPSTICK. Brace your little finger against your chin to keep your hand steady. If you want your lips to appear a bit fuller, apply a darker shade of lipstick with your lip liner first and fill in with a lighter shade. A wet, dewy look is needed and is easily obtained with a lip gloss. Gloss comes in a tube as well as in a case. You should not have to lick your lips to get this effect, as was done years ago, with chapped lips often the result. If you have very dry lips, there is a lip moisturizer that is excellent as an underbase. Check your current fashion magazines for the colors that seem best for you.

14. APPLY AN IRIDESCENT OVERBASE. Now that you've completed your makeup, the very last touch will be adding highlights of any dewy, iridescent touch. You definitely can use it under and around the outer eye area. Blend a drop around the eye. You may want a streak down your nose, a dab on the chin or forehead. Study the models in the magazines, and wherever you see shiny areas is where they have applied the iridescent overbase.

At this point your makeup is finished and you're ready for your assignment. Now, let me take you back to the special care and handling of your eyebrows. After you've learned all about shape and proportion, as well as the art of making them up, you can check the complete makeup—step by step—through the photographs that follow.

Eyebrows

We should think of our eyebrows as a frame. Your eyes are a picture, and the frame must be balanced or the picture is not perfect. Therefore, your brows must be spaced and suited to your bone structure, to the way your eyes are shaped on your face, the length of your nose, the width and height of your eyes. All these things are important to the effect of beautiful eyes.

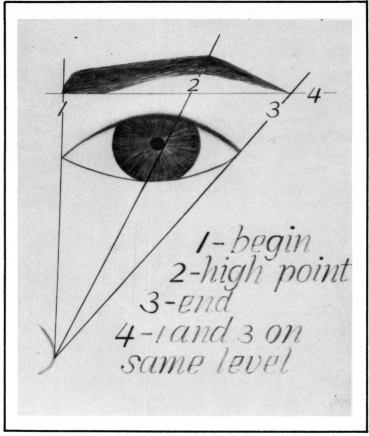

1- begin
2- high point
3- end
4- 1 and 3 on same level

Here is a perfect picture for you to follow in measuring your brow. Check your four points carefully.

By rights, the length of the eye from one corner to the other corner is the actual length of the eye. If you measure it, it should be the same as the width across the bridge of the nose from one eye to the other. In other words, it would be as if three eyes could be situated there, the original two and enough space for another eye in the center. This is what we call a perfectly spaced eye, but we'd like you to be very familiar with five different points and effects that brows can give. These are extremes we want to make sure you don't affect.

1. SHARP RISE FROM INNER CORNER. This will lengthen the nose and draw the eyes closer together, especially when you look at a brow and two of them close in.

2. PRONOUNCED DOWNWARD CURVE AT OUTER CORNER. This gives a sadder and older look. Any downward line is not good — either inner or outer — but this one gives a very sad and old look.

3. HIGH, ROUND "OWL" BROW. This gives a surprised look. Notice that when you raise your eyebrows, you round them out a bit. Lucille Ball is an example of this rather owlish appearance of the brow; she always has a surprised look. I frequently feel her brows were designed this way purposely because she is a comedienne and this look is good for her. For specific purposes, yes, but this effect is not wanted for a beautifully balanced look.

4. EXTREME UPWARD SLANT. This gives an Oriental look, and should be avoided.

5. HEAVY, SQUARE BEGINNING OF BROW/AND RATHER STRAIGHT BROW. This gives a masculine, angry look. If you were to look into a mirror now and frown, you'd notice that your eyebrows go straighter. There should be a gentle arch, to give a gentle youthfulness to the face.

Do not tweeze the top portion of the brow, though there are exceptions. If there is definitely a stray hair or the brows do not balance out, a few hairs may be tweezed occasionally. Generally speaking, though, tweeze and concentrate on the underside of the brow and between the eyes.

ITEMS NEEDED FOR BROW CARE

1. Cream — to soften the skin and make plucking easier.
2. Alcohol or freshener — to remove oil so that you can grasp hairs more easily.
3. Tweezers — the type is optional, but we like the slanted-edge, scissors type best. Always check tweezers when you buy them to make sure that the edges are even and close together, or that the tweezers haven't been dropped and are out of alignment. Be careful that you don't drop your tweezers.
4. Brush-comb for brow. Use a mascara brush, if you wish, but it isn't as good as the one specially designed for brows. Brows need combing and brushing just as your hair does; the skin flakes, and brows should be done daily.
5. Brush-on for darkening. We prefer a brush if darkening is needed — and with most brows, it is. It should be done with a brush-on rather than a pencil. Pencils contain oil and give a harsher look. Darken only the area where needed. If hair is very blonde, darkening would be needed. In most cases, it is only necessary to fill in areas and balance the picture of the brow. Don't put it on your hair.
6. Coloring. Your brows should be the same color as your hair or lighter, and today the trend is lighter. There are items on the market

that you can brush on to give a softer, blonder look to your brows. Sometimes girls bleach them. If you have blond hair, your eyebrows should be light.

We suggest that girls look for a picture of brows that look like their own, and keep it with their makeup. Place it where you will look at it and compare it with your own brows every day. You'd be surprised. There are many different brows on models. You will find one type that's right for you. Once you achieve good brows, they are one of the easiest areas to skip. You can start off right, and then forget about your eyebrows. This is why we suggest that you measure your brows regularly to be sure you're doing them correctly.

HOW TO SHAPE YOUR EYEBROWS

I'd like you to actually draw a picture. Once you draw a picture, you can better understand my instructions. Taking a pencil to measure your brow from the side of your nose — starting at the lower edge of the nostril, it would be a straight line from it to the beginning line of your brow. Then hold the pencil from the edge of the nostril to the outer corner of your eye, and that would be the ending of the brow. Put a little dot to mark the spot. Take your pencil and put a little point; beginning and then the end. Now stare straight into the mirror, take your pencil and rest it along the outside edge of the pupil — so that you can see — and put a little dot at the top of the brow. You usually can see fine little hairs; this is where your high point should be. It gives a lift to your face.

You don't want to neglect the high point of your brow. It is not at the beginning, but at the outer edge of the pupil. Your fourth line is a very important line. You place a pencil from the beginning of the brow, straight across to the end of the brow, and you should have a straight line. The beginning and ending of the brows should be on a straight line. You don't want that outer edge to be below the line, or the beginning edge. It is all on a straight line. The arch comes up in the center, as you can see.

How much space comes between and in through the shadowing area is determined by the width of your eyes and the way your brows grow, but you must see skin from the left eye to the right eye. This space should be clear so that you get an open look to the eyes. Approximately the width of the center of your eye — the full width of your eye — is about the same space as you would have from the corners to the beginning of your brow.

Your eyebrows should be brushed and combed. If you have curly ones, and this sometimes happens, they can be straightened with moustache wax. Some of the hair gels, if used strongly and pressed on every night, will help to straighten them, but excess curl can be controlled by combing and brushing. Some girls who have a slight curl tame the brows with very heavy Vaseline. I think that hair-setting solutions and gels are better.

Now, after you've measured your brows and brushed them in — or even penciled them in — you start to tweeze. If you hold the skin taut, by taking two fingers and stretching the skin, always pulling the hair in the direction you want it to grow, you'll find that hairs are apt to grow in the way you pull them. Any stray hairs should be tweezed daily. This is important. Don't wait all week to do your brows for a once-a-week ritual. This should be as automatic as putting on lipstick. Look in your magnifying mirror and see if there are any stray hairs across the bridge of your nose or a stray one that may have grown down into an area where it shouldn't be. Hair grows in different lengths. Once brows are shaped properly, it's never a major job to attend to them every day. You don't keep a job as a model if your photographs show unsightly hairs growing!

Tweeze your eyebrows every single day. I think this is something that isn't stressed enough. Do it even if it's only one hair. There may not be any, but be sure to check. It's best to pluck strays after you have brushed your brows, so that you won't take a chance of removing too many hairs. If you start making them thinner, then you're very apt to go astray. You can see what's necessary after you've brushed, especially getting up close to your brow line. Then you won't go off it.

Measure them constantly to double-check. Keep them soft and light. Your eyebrows should have a clean look. In some cases, photography models are gifted with enough clearly defined brows so that they don't need any brush-on, but in most cases a girl will need a little bit at the tail end to balance the picture. If she measures her brows and they come out beautifully, fine. But if she needs a little tinge of height — sometimes hair is a little fine on the upper high point — she'll need to color that end a bit, but never have a harsh look on the brow.

As with all our makeup tips, you will need practice and patience. Be conscientious, and practice constantly until you're practically picture-perfect. Now, turn the pages and you'll see how Dick and Carlo La Torre have taken a model through all the stages of an ideal makeup session — from a well-scrubbed start to a glamorous finish. Study the makeup and brows of every model in this book.

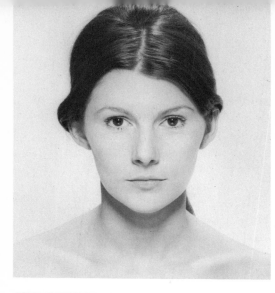

Here's our model before the magic of a skillful makeup. Her skin has been thoroughly cleansed with Cream Float and freshened with a skin freshener. Now she's ready for the work to begin. She's pretty now, but just wait!

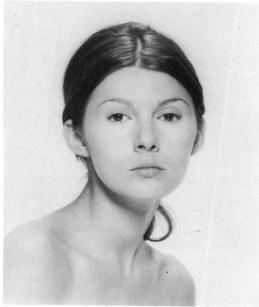

T. V. Touch is smoothed on under eyes to blend out circles and cover blemishes.

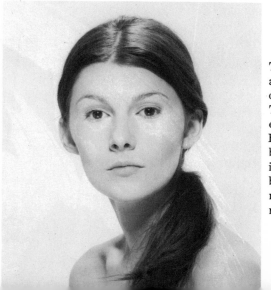

The four steps that bring us to this stage are: 1. Makeup foundation applied with dry foam sponge over entire face and T. V. Touch. 2. Translucent powder dusted over foundation with powder brush. 3. Rouge brush used to apply rouge on cheekbone area. 4. Blond shading below rouge in hollow cheekbone area with contour brush, also applied lightly on sides of nose to make it look perfect. Fluff brush may be used for nose area.

To bring out the beauty of her eyes: 1. Brush on eyebrows. 2. Gray-brown eye shadow applied with shadow brush to create a contour under eyebone. 3. Toast eye shadow to highlight under brow and on eyelid with wide, flat brush.

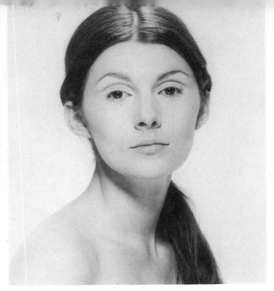

Brown eyeliner with liner seal along the base of the lashes. Thin line and small extension only.

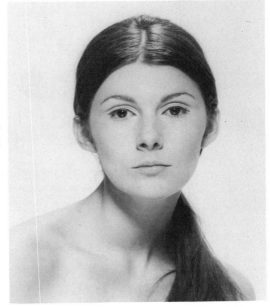

A small amount of fluid mascara is applied to the upper lashes. The brown contour line will vary according to your bone and eye structure. Sometimes wider and less defined by applying with a fluff brush.

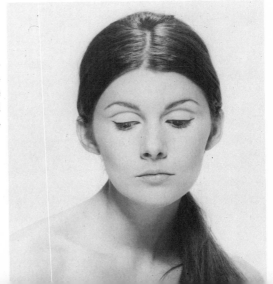

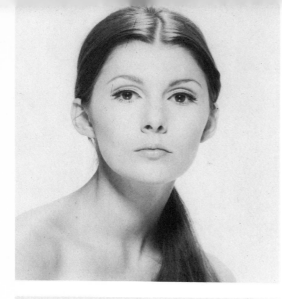

Brown false lashes are applied with surgical glue. Mascara brushed on both false and natural lashes. Models should have a variety of lashes for different assignments.

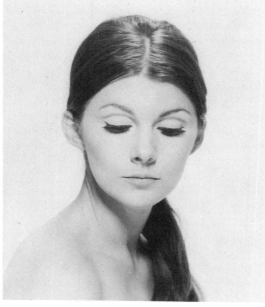

Looking at our model from a different angle, you can see the precise shaping in every detail of this eye makeup. Perfect for her eyes.

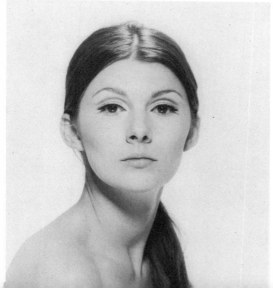

Last to go on is the lipstick. Use a brush for the outline and fill in with an iridescent lip gloss for color and depth.

Here she is, radiant in a complete makeup which has been perfectly plotted and magnificently carried out. Isn't she beautiful?

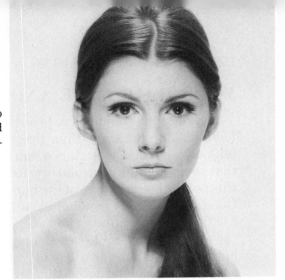

Our model is surrounded by her complete collection of Dick and Carlo La Torre's "Onstage" makeup—everything she'll need to cover any makeup situation. Notice the wide variety of brushes, so important to the proper application of different cosmetics with their different textures and needs.

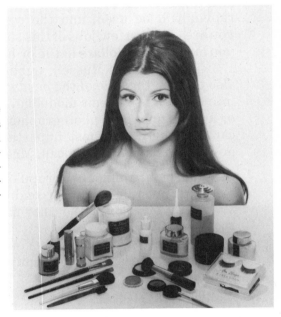

Here top fashion model Ellen Harth of the Frances Gill Model Agency shows what an artist she is with her own creation. Not every model can be this extreme, but you practice and practice to be an individual. Your makeup must mean something to your face.

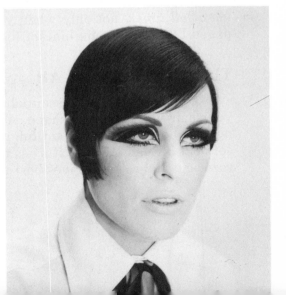

YOUR HAIR CARE AND WIG WARDROBE

Every girl should have beautiful hair, but a successful model *must* have it. More reasons than the obvious one are involved. Modeling for hair products, for instance, can often be a convenient way to acquire that so-important portfolio of photographs. Indispensable to a model, this portfolio can be one of the most expensive items in her equipment. Good photography is never cheap, and if your photos aren't taken by a skilled photographer, they are no use to you at all.

It is often possible to do hair-product modeling—if you're a beginner—in exchange for a set of photographs for yourself. Since we'll assume that you're doing this for a firm that wants its products displayed to the best possible advantage, you can be sure that a top photographer will be used, and the resultant pictures perfect. So, there you are—after a few jobs of this sort—with a portfolio that would cost you hundreds of dollars in the ordinary way.

Terry Grimes Russell, publicity manager for Clairol, Inc., will also tell you that one of the best ways for a beginning model to break into the field is via hair modeling. This can be for a hair-product firm, or a magazine, or a photographer. Whichever you're aiming for, we caution, there are most important basic requirements. When you go out on a hair-modeling call, Mrs. Russell suggests:

1. You hair must be scrupulously clean and shining.
2. It must be in superb condition and have sufficient body.
3. If you color it, the color must always be even; no other-color roots ever!
4. Don't use hair spray. Your hair should have enough body to make it unnecessary. If you must use spray, just a fine, light mist will do.
5. Don't argue with the hairdresser. He's the star here, not you.

Above all, your hair must be strong, healthy, vigorous, and gleaming *at all times,* not only when you go out on call. In the following pages, I'll give you some hints on hair care that should be very helpful.

The Kindest Cut of All

A good basic cut is essential. Even when the setting comes out, your hair will retain its shape. At worst, your hair will always look neat; at best, it will be beautiful. If your hair is very fine, a blunt-scissors cut is best. If the texture is medium to coarse, a combination of razor-cut and scissors gives best results—the razor to taper the hair and the scissors for a final shaping. If your hair is very fine, a layered cut isn't always a happy choice, unless you're proficient with nightly sets and have the patience—and time!—to indulge in them. For fine hair, a blunt cut, which is all one length, would be the answer. This would give maximum body.

Of course, your best bet—and there's really no way out of this—is to find yourself a skillful hair stylist who can give you an ideal basic cut. This isn't always easy, but it's almost certain that any town or city large enough to have modeling jobs would also be sophisticated enough to have at least one good stylist. Find him! Or her! With your basic cut, all you'll need will be a little patience and practice and you'll be able to handle setting chores yourself.

Some hair stylists can do a cut that will last from six to eight weeks. This is a boon to the busy model and a blessing to the one who is going on a location assignment. Did you know that hair has a tendency to grow faster from different sections of the scalp? A stylist should study his client, learn the pattern, and then compensate in the overgrowing areas. If the back of your hair grows faster, only the neckline and back are trimmed; if it grows faster at the crown, the hair at the nape is left longer.

To be considered along with your cut: If your hair is too curly for your taste, it must be straightened, and if, conversely, it falls apart right after a set, it may need a body wave.

Choosing Your Best Hairstyles

The very fact that you're a model makes it imperative for you to have, and be able to wear, a variety of hairstyles. Your hairpieces will be a big help here, and we'll go into more detail on that later, but here are some tips on choosing the styles that are right for you.

So many articles and books on hairstyling say that you should choose a style according to the shape of your face. Forget it. This concept simply isn't true any more. A contemporary hairstyle no longer must attempt to make your face look oval. If it does, of course, so much the better. What we do want, though, is a hairdo that says something that is *you*. A hairstyle that gives you a definite personality or, better yet, interprets your own personality.

You can take any hairstyle at all and apply it to any type of girl and—with a few personal adjustments—suit it to her particular shape of face, her way of life, or her specific age group.

How do you choose a hairstyle?

Find the hairdo that is "in"—the hairdo of the moment. I don't mean the most extreme style you can find, though occasionally you may have to wear one for a special modeling job. Adopt the chic, shapely new styles, and you needn't worry about looking like everybody else because hairdos can be modified or altered to enhance the individual. Choosing a hairstyle of the moment means that you must always be aware of new trends, new ideas, new concepts in beauty styles as well as fashion.

Unless the mood of a hairstyle is an especially smooth and finished one, it should always have a light and airy look about it. Don't choose a hairdo that will be difficult to manage and care for if you're not the handy type.

Hair trends, of course, are widely variable. Sometimes a fad or fancy will last for a long time, until it's literally pushed out by an entirely new look, but usually changes come fast and often. You have to be constantly aware of them, and be ready for them all the time.

One thing that seems to run through all the trends, in any year, is emphasis on the shape of the head. Except for the years of the madly exaggerated bouffants, most hairdos basically follow the lines of the head, which, again, proves the importance of a good haircut. For a long time, too, hairstyles were partless. Well, little by little, the part has been creeping back into hair designs and, while not picked up by every stylist, will probably never fade back into oblivion.

The style that features a part brings with it an attendant hazard. Hair color must be absolutely perfect, or that parting can really be "sweet sorrow!" No more camouflaging those dark roots by brushing up and over, even if the partings are partial, misted, or diagonal. If the part shows at all, even glimmers through, the color must be flawless.

For any style, hair has to be sleek and shining as well as skillfully shaped. It has to be cleaned and brushed, and regularly conditioned. It has to have body and swing and bounce. You'll have to learn to make it that way, and keep it that way.

On the following pages you will see a number of beautiful hairstyles by leading stylists, each illustrating a different principle of shaping and design. All from Clairol, two of the hairdos—a short and a mid-length—are accompanied by detailed setting patterns. Choose the ones you think would be right for you, then read on and learn how to keep your hair lovely enough to wear them.

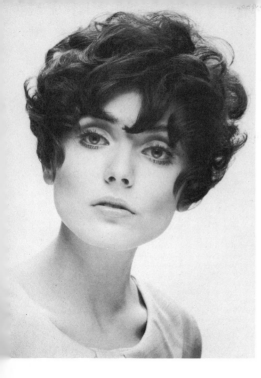

Hollywood's Gene Shacove designed this free and easy short cut. Curled and care-free, it's an ideal short styling for features which tend to be square.

All hair style photos by Philip E. Pegler except where noted.

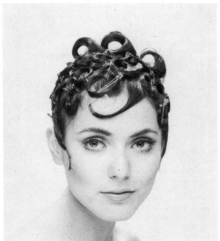

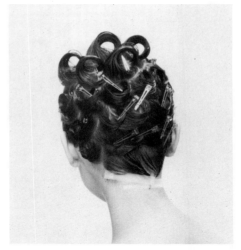

This hairdo uses only pincurls and Scotch tape, no rollers at all. Pincurls at the crown are the stand-up type; the rest are flat. Long strand in front and one on both sides are gently curved and anchored with Scotch tape. Short hair at nape is also Scotch taped. Exclusive use of pincurls is best for a short, curly do like this.

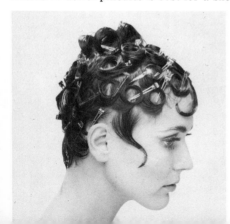

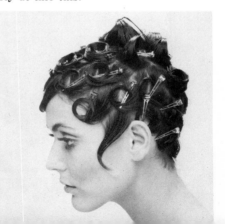

Delightfully demure, this caplike coif by Daniel of New York's Saks Fifth Avenue features a brief part and lightly ruffled ends. This is good for a wide oval face or an almost round one.

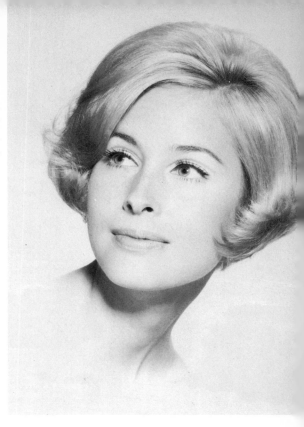

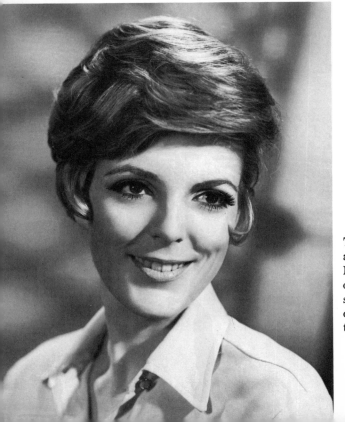

This short hairdo is by Leslie Blanchard, a master colorist as well as a brilliant New York stylist. This is good for a long oval face with pointed jawline. Notice soft curls on cheek and special effects created with the use of a frost-and-tip technique.

Photo by Bud Fraker

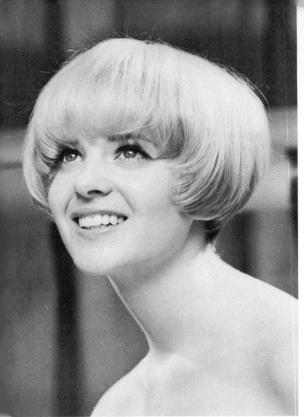

Here's a gay little hairdo by Mr. Zorro. It's for an oval face, though it could look well on a slightly rounded one if the features are good, and the wearer quite young. It is preferable that your brows show for expression.

Photo by Herb Brewer

This unique and exquisite design is by French stylist Jean Marc Elrhodes. No compromise here, this is for the perfect oval only.

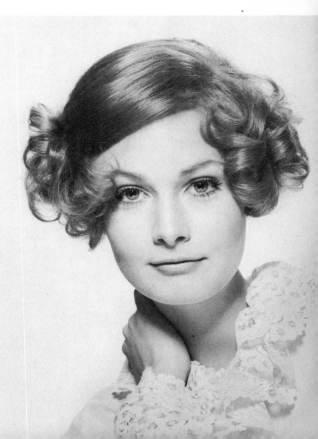

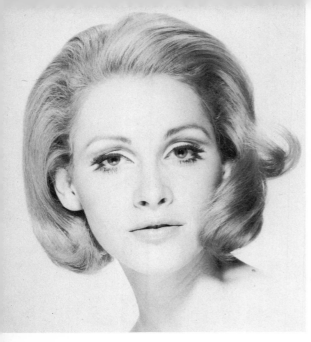

This soft mid-length hairstyle was created by Anthony Migliaro of the Joyce Christopher Beauty Salon in New York. A pretty face-framing style for anyone, the rounder the face, the greater the height.

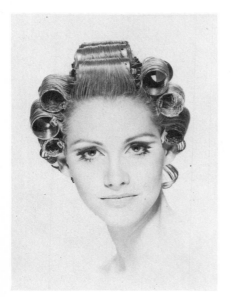 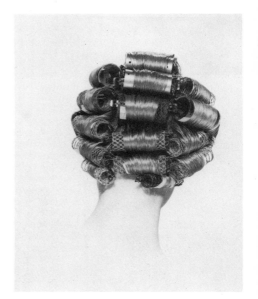

All rollers are used for this style. The 3 sizes involved are (1) Large at top and front, (2) medium at back and above ears, and (3) small at the nape. Rollers best achieve the smooth, buoyant effect for a mid-length style like this.

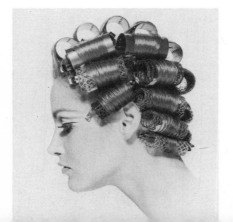 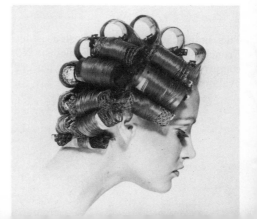

Hugh Harrison styles this mid-length do for an oval or a widened, almost round, oval. You can break the width with a wave.

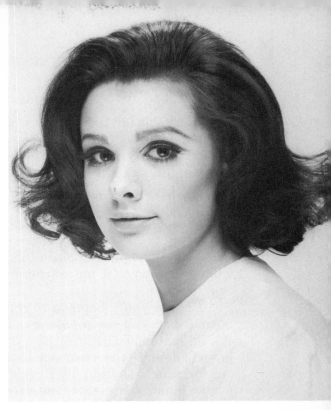

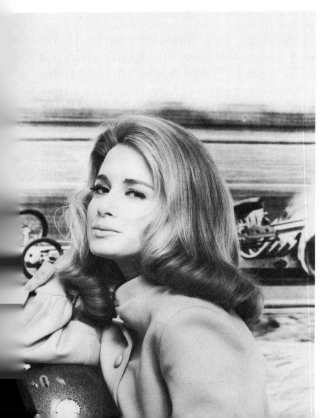

Our one really long hairstyle is by Paul Mitchell of Henri Bendel in New York. It's perfect for a pear-shaped face, as a prominent jaw can be minimized with a deep wave at the jawline.

Photo by Sam Joasten

Pamper Your Hair

You can't fail to keep your hair in a perpetual glow if you'll just remember three things: 1. Keep it clean. 2. Brush it daily. 3. Condition it regularly. All of these have to be done the right way, or you're wasting your time.

SHAMPOOING TIPS

What *not* to do is to shampoo your hair according to schedule. Not every week, or every three days, or whenever. Wash your hair every time it begins to look dull and feels oily. Blondes and city dwellers will need to wash it more frequently than brunettes who live in the country.

Choose your shampoo to conform to the type of your hair. For normal hair, you can get along quite nicely with any neutral shampoo. A mild shampoo with an oil base is a must for dry hair, otherwise washing will deplete the natural hair oils. For oily hair, you'll need a vigorous formula to thoroughly cleanse the hair and remove all the oil. Always a bland shampoo for tinted or lightened hair. Ordinary shampoos will affect the color and, fortunately, there are several color-keyed formulas on the market that will keep your color as true as possible.

Once you've settled on the type of shampoo you need—and, oddly enough, this can change from time to time with varying circumstances—you should know how to use it. I know, anyone should know how to wash her hair. It's elementary—right? Wrong. You'll get better results if you do it correctly.

Give your hair one or two sudsings; two, if it's very dirty. If you live in a hard-water area, use a water softener. Distribute shampoo thoroughly by pouring it into the palms of your hands, rubbing them together, and then smoothing them over your wet hair. Work the lather into your scalp with your fingertips, using a circular motion, and don't neglect the hairline. This is especially important at the forehead and doubly true if you're in the habit of wearing bangs.

Of course, avoid extremes of water temperature, since too-hot water can remove necessary oil or oversoften the hair strands. Cold water can be a shock to the scalp and can sometimes cause headaches, though if you use gradually cooling water as you rinse, your hair will have more body. Lukewarm water is just right for washing, cool off as you rinse, and your final rinse can be with cold water.

Be sure to penetrate clear through to your scalp when you rinse; it would pay to invest in an inexpensive rubber shower spray for this. Rinse until the water runs clear. If you're a blonde, a lemon rinse is great; brunettes can get the same effect with a vinegar rinse.

Pat or blot your hair dry with your towel. Be gentle, as vigorous rubbing encourages tangles and could break brittle ends. If you're using an electric dryer, don't use it at high heat or for an extended time; either process is likely to dry out your hair and your scalp. A good idea, incidentally, while you're under the dryer, would be to apply moisturizing cream to your face to prevent your skin from drying out.

CONDITIONING

Some hair takes special handling, and this is especially true in a model's life, where she has to work under hot lights, glaring sun, wind, and all kinds of weather. This means conditioning is in order. Ordinary hair will need conditioning, too, but the new "instant" conditioners will be ample. For special treatment of hair that's been overexposed to sunlight and hot lights, here's a routine that won't be too difficult to follow and will do worlds of good.

Section off your hair in one-inch partings and dab conditioner or warm olive oil all over your scalp, using your fingertips or a bit of cotton. Then cover your hair with hot towels and let it "rest" for a while before you shampoo. Then shampoo, following the suggestions above.

Note: Coarse hair needs a softening shampoo and a cream rinse to make it easier to handle. Very fine hair must have a soapless shampoo that contains oils and a conditioner for body. A cream rinse is absolutely taboo for this type of hair, or it will become completely unmanageable.

The Way to a Smart Set

It hardly seems possible that any young girl doesn't know how to set her hair these days. In fact, many of the resultant stylings look absolutely professional. But, just in case the mechanics of do-it-yourself hair setting have escaped you until now, here's a brief rundown of an easy routine. Be sure you learn it. If there's one thing a busy model will have to know, it's how to do her own hair in a pinch. She may be stuck on location in the heart of a desert or at the bottom of a canyon — really, it has happened! — with the nearest hairdresser hundreds of miles away. This could spell total disaster, but not if you know how to set your own hair.

Set hair good and damp, unless you have to dry it in a great hurry or want a very loose set. (If you're using one of the new electric roller sets, then your hair should be towel-dried only and the wetness kept to a minimum.) Usually hair responds better when it is well dampened and it will have less of a tendency to be frizzy or dry looking when combed out. Choice of a setting medium is up to you, according to your own preference. If your hair is limp, use one of the conditioner setting lotions that give such great body and sheen to the hair.

Rollers should be used for most of the setting, but with short hair it is sometimes necessary to put sections of it into pincurls, particularly above the ear and at the nape line. Again, it's a matter of being aware of the trend of the moment. For the very curly coifs that crop up from time to time, you would use more pincurls than rollers. Some of these hairdos won't require rollers at all.

ABOUT PINCURLS. There are two techniques for pincurling. For a softer curl, hair is rolled from its tip toward the scalp or around the tip of the finger. For a tighter set or firmer curl, hair is rolled from the root out.

ABOUT ROLLERS. Use larger rollers for top and crown; medium ones for sides and back; and narrower ones for the nape. It depends, of course, on the length of hair, its texture, and the result desired. The amount of hair for each roller should equal the width of the roller and be slightly less than the length of the roller. Do roll smoothly and keep hair taut. Zigzagging the parting will keep hair from separating when combed out.

The Comb-out

When dry, your hair should be brushed out very thoroughly. Use a firm brush and—if you can get one—a brush with a combination of natural and nylon bristles. This combines the strength of the nylon with the added natural bristle properties of being able to distribute the oils through the hair, thus reducing static electricity.

If you can possibly brush in front of an open window or outdoors in good weather, this will be most beneficial. Also, it is good to bend forward from the waist and brush with your head hanging down. This stimulates the flow of blood to the scalp.

When your hair has been thoroughly brushed, you can brush it into whatever lines you wish. I mean, naturally, lines which are compatible with your setting pattern.

Back-combing or some teasing of the hair is sometimes necessary to give it form and body, especially at the top and crown area. Two methods can be used. One is back-combing with a comb; the other with a brush. The comb usually gives a firmer base, and the brush gives a lighter and airier look to your hair.

Holding the hair strand up firmly, it is back-combed lightly in short strokes starting from the base of the hair and working up toward the tips of the strand. Don't do this carelessly or roughly, as this can mat and tear your hair. The idea is to make a cushion at the scalp which will lift the hair away from the head, giving it fullness and form, and leave the ends free to give it smoothness or curl. At the hairline, don't bring the comb through the strand or it will be difficult to smooth over to hide the teasing.

Finish up by spraying lightly. Use the most natural-looking hair spray you can find, unless you're modeling in a highly intricate coif that has to be actually lacquered. In any case, you probably wouldn't be handling a hairdo like this yourself; this is almost strictly the province of the professional hairdresser. When using the spray, hold the can at least 6 to 8 inches away from your hair and move it constantly as you use it. You'll get a much softer and natural-looking hold this way.

To Color or Not

If you're not really happy with the hair color you already have, by all means change it. Whether the resulting difference is slight enough so that "only your hairdresser will know," or bold enough to give you an entirely new look, it's what it does to your self-confidence that really counts. The merest addition of a sparkling highlight can make you feel secure and confident. A mousy brown can go to a gleaming chestnut with just a touch of a temporary rinse. Or you might want a change more dramatic than that. You can go from a nondescript brown to a glorious sunlit blonde. It's a complete change, but maybe you were meant to be a blonde all along! Now your hair color goes with your personality.

Of course, you may be perfectly satisfied with your natural hair color, and all you have to do is keep it clean and sparkling. If, however, you do decide to change it, do so with assurance. More women than ever before are changing their hair color, and with as little self-consciousness as wearing false lashes.

There are a few things you should know about hair coloring before you decide it's for you. First of all, there are some things you can do yourself and some you can't. You *can:* (1) Give yourself any of the temporary rinses. (2) Lighten your hair if it's already a natural shade of blonde. (3) Color your hair in any of the brunettes, and some of the reds and darker blondes. You *shouldn't:* (1) Attempt any of the tricky techniques like tipping, frosting, or streaking. (2) Do any coloring that requires two processes such as blonding that calls for stripping first. Yes, there are quick and comparatively easy toners on the market that you can use, and they generally work well, but your good looks are your working equipment and you can't afford to take chances.

If you're planning to change your hair color for the first time, it's always a good idea to have it done professionally, whether you're planning a drastic change or a switch of a shade or two. Then you can decide whether you'll be able to go on with it yourself. Regular touchups, of course, are an absolute must. According to Clairol's Terry Russell, it's unbelievable how many professional models will arrive for a hair-modeling interview with dark roots showing! Naturally they don't get the job, but it seems difficult to understand how a professional can make such a mistake. Don't you make it.

On Location

You should be ready for small emergencies whenever you go out on an assignment, and you should always carry a small brush, comb, and miniature hairspray in your model's kit. When you go off on location, though, you'll need more. As I mentioned before, it's just possible that you may be working in an area where no hair stylist is available. Besides knowing how to handle your own hair in a pinch, you should have the materials on hand that will make this easier for you. Famous New York hair stylist Hugh Harrison—whose clientele consists mainly of socialites and top models—has made up a list of haircare equipment for his "jet set" clients to take with them when they travel. Here it is:

1. The right shampoo.
2. One of the double-duty formulas that conditions and sets.
3. A brush or comb for styling, according to individual preference.
4. One of the new electric roller kits for a fast set and comb-out.
5. A softening agent, in case your itinerary takes you to a hard-water area.
6. A miniature can of hairspray.

Hugh also suggests that you take along a variety of hairpieces. An easy way to pack them, he finds, is to set them, roll them up on the cardboard rollers that are inside paper towels, then tuck them into your bag.

Yes, you definitely must have hairpieces. You could possibly start out with one or two and eventually work up to a whole wardrobe of spare hair goods. It will be a worthwhile investment, and just wait until you see all the wonderful things you can do with them!

Your Wig Wardrobe

At the beginning, your wardrobe will actually consist of hairpieces. There are many types of hairpieces, but you would probably be ready for almost any assignment if you owned a wiglet, a braid, and a fall. Incidentally, until you learn how to handle hairpieces, I'd suggest you use the synthetic kind. They're less expensive than human hair (important when you're just starting out!) and are easier to work with.

THE WIGLET

A wiglet must be the same color as your own hair, unless you're deliberately trying for an unusual effect. It can be anchored high at the crown, tilted to one side, low at the back near the nape, or high at the back of the crown. It depends on you and the effect you are striving for. It should be attached securely with hairpins.

THE BRAID

You can call it a braid, or a ponytail, or a chignon. Actually, it's a long hank of hair that you can shape into all sorts of auxiliaries. Basically, your braid should be the same shade as your own hair, but you can get some exciting effects if you have an extra one just a shade or two lighter or darker. This piece is about the easiest to put on. Once you've braided it, or plaited it, or styled it the way you want, all you do is pin it on, generally high at the crown or low at the side.

THE FALL

The fall—occasionally called a demi-wig—comes in many lengths, but basically it is a luxuriant length of hair that falls straight from a tiny caplike foundation. Like the wiglet and braid, it should be in your own hair color. You can wear your fall exactly as it is and let it swing casually loose, or you can have it elaborately styled. It can be styled in loops, clusters, waves, or curls. It can be an elegant upsweep or a cascade of curls. It depends on your hairdresser or—if you're handy with a hairdo—on you. A fall is usually attached to a small, square base about 2 inches by 2 inches, and you can anchor it securely to your head with the aid of properly placed hairpins.

THE SINGLE CURL

Now you can buy still another type of hair goods, the single curl. You can buy it singly or in clusters, and just simply add the single curls onto your coiffure wherever you think they'll look best. Get some in your natural hair color and—for special effects—some in a contrasting hue.

THE FULL WIG

This is the one you'll get last of all, when you're getting more bookings (and are, consequently, richer). Your first wig should be the color of your own hair, so that you can use it when you don't have time to have your hair set or colored. You can even, if you're skillful, blend a full wig with your own hair. When you get your second wig, you can go into another color or style. Full wigs come in a variety of lengths, from a long, elaborately styled design to the gay little mini stretch wigs.

Your best bet in learning to apply your wig is to watch your stylist. Briefly, this is the way you do it. If your hair is long, you must get it well out of the way before you put on your wig. The best way to do this is to make large, flat pincurls all over your head. Then apply your wig and fasten it securely to the pincurls with hairpins. Your wig, of course, must be fitted *exactly* to your head. If your hair is short, all you have to do is smooth your hair back, and pin it up and away from your face so that it won't show.

Your hairpieces should be properly stored in their own containers, when you're not using them. You can wash the synthetic pieces, but human hair must be dry-cleaned. Unless you're very, very skillful, I'd advise you to have your human hair goods cleaned and styled by your hairdresser.

You can get styling ideas for your wigs and hairpieces from your hairdresser and from the fashion magazines. There are some marvelous styling ideas in the hairdo magazines, too, but if you'll look at the following pages you'll see some beautiful and ingenious designs for hairpieces that were done for us by Enny of Italy.

Enny is one of the most brilliant hair stylists, here and abroad, and an undisputed genius of the art of the wigmaker. Winner of numerous awards in Italy, France, and America and longtime director of the annual International Hairdressers' Show in New York, Enny creates hairstyles for socialites, film and stage stars, and leading models.

Falls come in several lengths. This is mid-length and is made to appear shorter by styling with a lift at the crown. Ends have a semi-pageboy effect.

Wig photos by Enny of Italy

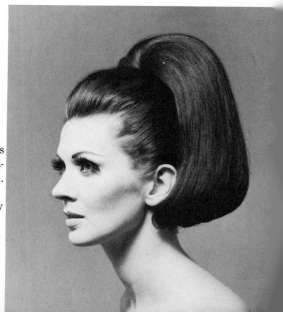

A long fall, this one is styled with flipped-up ends that just skim the shoulders. The crisscross strands of hair serve two purposes—as a decorative accent and to mask the joining line of natural hair and fall. These strands can be worked either with your own hair or that of the fall.

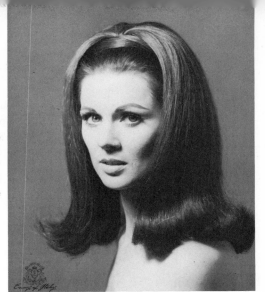

Another—more sophisticated—way to wear a long fall is to anchor it farther back at the crown, where twisted hair strands are fuller, thicker, and raised to give height to the hairdo. Ears are bared for this style.

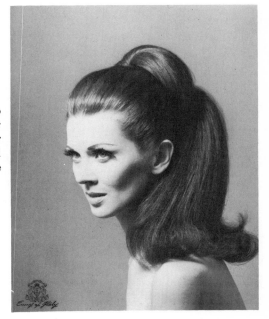

This elegant and formal styling is achieved with a hairpiece. It can also be done with two hairpieces; one for the spiral curl down the back and one for the double coil atop the crown. If you're very good with your hair, you can use a long fall for this.

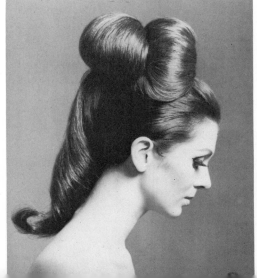

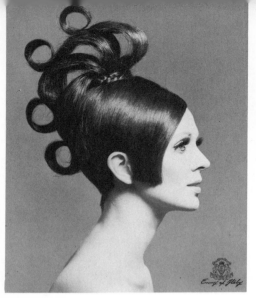

Strictly for gala evening costumes, this do features a hairpiece that's intricately styled in an arrangement of strategically placed loops and curls.

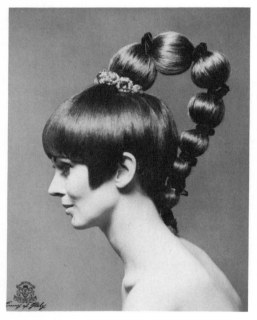

Here's a definitely different way to handle a ponytail. A hairdo like this is also a partygoer but would be so much more at home with fun party clothes. You can get this effect by tucking styrofoam balls in graduated sizes at intervals in the ponytail and tying each one with ribbon. Attach the piece high on the crown. Short hair on the model is her own, but if yours is long, just wear a short wig with the ponytail.

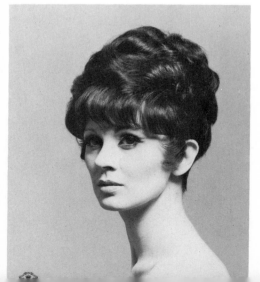

Finally, we have the mini stretch wig, Enny's creation. It's a light and airy little wig ingeniously designed to slip comfortably over your own hair. Easy to manage, it can be styled in dozens of delightful ways.

YOUR FIGURE

You can still be a fashion model if your face isn't perfectly beautiful, but you won't be able to find a place in the field if your figure isn't good. No matter what size range you fit into, your figure must be trim and attractive so that you'll look well in the clothes you're showing.

Contrary to popular belief, all models aren't naturally thin. While it's true that many of them are, with some even having to eat to keep up their weight, an equal number have to work at keeping their weight down to where they want it.

If you adopt sensible eating habits and a simple exercise routine now, you'll never have to worry about your figure. There's no point in getting complicated and going into all sorts of fancy exercises and crash diets. Here are some simple pointers that should help you to get—and keep—the weight that is ideal for you.

Diet

You should always have balanced regular meals. Don't skip any of the three you need every day. You can add snacks, but they must be the nonfattening kind. If you have a tendency to gain, weigh yourself every day. Never gain more than two pounds. When you do, it's time to diet.

Be sensible about your eating habits. You need protein, some carbohydrates, green vegetables, fruit (at least one citrus), and milk or a milk product every day. If you're slimming, stick to the leafy green vegetables and stay away from the starchy ones. Get yourself a calorie chart (or a little booklet you can carry with you) and learn which foods have the least calories and are good for you.

You always need protein, whether you're dieting or not. A good way to determine how much protein you need is to divide your weight by two. The resulting number shows how many protein grams you need for your minimum daily requirement. A model should eat extra protein for protection.

This is not a book on nutrition, so I'm not going into all kinds of diets and food facts. What I want to do is convince you to eat sensibly and get into good eating habits. Here is a sample slimming diet that has worked very well for our girls. If you want to go into this more thoroughly, you can read up on nutrition in your library.

SAMPLE DIET

Breakfast
  4 oz. juice *or* ½ grapefruit

1 egg
½ slice of toast;
1 pat margarine, if needed
(If you're in a hurry,
beat your egg into
the juice.)

Lunch
¼ cup cottage cheese
1 medium tomato
        or
Salad of greens
        or
Vegetable soup (8 oz.)
2 crackers

Dinner
3 oz. lean meat broiled, no sauces
Green vegetables, no butter or sauces
Salad, diet dressing
Fruit, 1 fresh or canned (diet pack)

Snacks: Celery, carrot sticks, spoonful of cottage cheese, diet drinks or diet gelatins to satisfy your sweet tooth.

Avoid: Potatoes, rice, corn, bread, desserts, candy, and large servings of anything.

Stick with this diet until you have reached your desired weight. Have small servings and don't skip any meals. Once you've reached the right weight, don't go overboard and eat everything in sight to celebrate! You'll only have to do it all over again, and the next time it may be more difficult.

Exercise

I think every model should exercise. Even if you don't have a weight problem, exercise will help your proportions, correct your posture, and give you a general feeling of health and well-being. Remember that exercise will *not reduce* your weight. It may reshape a curve or two, but only eating less will actually cause pounds to disappear.

Since each girl has different figure problems, I can't give you specific exercises here. Any good spot-reducing routines will do for special areas. As for posture, balance, and correct walking, you'll find my exercises for these in Chapter 3.

While the actual exercises will vary, there are certain rules which hold true for any type or method. Here they are; follow them to get the most out of your efforts.

EXERCISE RULES

1. Set aside a certain period each day for exercising. Any time of day is fine, except one hour after eating and when you are really tired.

2. Begin routine with milder exercises and stretching, as a warm-up before going on with more vigorous exercises.

3. It is not wise to exercise to the point of exhaustion, as the effects are considerably lessened when muscles are overworked. Rest for a few seconds between exercises, and pause between them if you think it is necessary.

4. If you find that exercising in two shifts is easier on you, do so. The results will be the same.

5. Although exercises should be performed moderately slowly, you shouldn't just go through the motions. Use your muscles and feel each exercise.

6. Always exercise on a mat, blanket, or rug. Be sure it doesn't skid or move.

7. When you have reached your ideal proportions, it is time to gradually decrease the number of figure exercises until you are doing just a few for general health and problem spots. Continually check your posture.

8. You may continue your exercises during your menstrual period; it is best to eliminate extreme twisting exercises at this time.

Make regular exercise so much a part of your daily living that it becomes second nature to you. If your figure is already perfect, just do toning and limbering routines. If it's a little less than perfect, check the parts of your body that need attention and concentrate on these.

Figure Analysis

Every model is different, but there are approximate measurements which are fairly general. Measurements for today's models run roughly along these lines:

Bust—32 through 34 inches.
Waist—21 through 24 or 25 inches.
Hips—from 33 to 36 inches.

Approximate weight would be:

Height	Model Weight
5 feet 5 inches	110 – 115 lbs.
5 feet 6 inches	110 – 118
5 feet 7 inches	110 – 121
5 feet 8 inches	115 – 124
5 feet 9 inches	118 – 127

You should know your exact measurements. For a perfect measuring chart, always lay tape flat over your body and don't pull it taut. These are your correct measuring points:

Bust — Be certain tape is straight across back.
Waist — Smallest area above hipbone.
Upper hip — Over hipbone and tummy.
Lower hip — Measure over largest portion of hips.
Upper thigh — Over top, heaviest part.
Lower thigh — Halfway between knee and upper thigh.
Knee — Measure just above knee bone.
Calf — Largest area about midway between knee and ankle.
Ankle — Above anklebone.
Wrist — Over wristbone.

Take these measurements when you're at your ideal weight, keep a chart of them, and try to keep them constant at all times.

YOUR GROOMING

Your hair is shining and stunningly styled, you have a flawless skin with a perfect makeup, your figure is great, your clothes are chic and a marvelous fit. The picture is complete. But is it?

Not if your grooming is careless. Meticulous grooming would seem to be elementary — especially for someone planning a career in modeling — but it is amazing how many girls sin in the opposite direction. So very many of them are well-turned-out on the surface and utterly slipshod about the little things. Like using a good deodorant, or trimming a hangnail, or keeping a shoulder strap up where it belongs.

After all, you're trying to sell yourself. The final, salable you is the *total* you, the final product after scrupulous attention to every trivial detail of grooming. It's all of you that counts, and here are some pointers to help you to that total beauty.

The Bath

You can tackle a number of grooming problems during your bath. Of course, a shower is handy and quick and wonderful when you're in a hurry, but there's nothing like a leisurely bath to keep you in the pink of perfection. Try to fit a regular bath into your schedule, no matter how crowded and hectic that schedule may be. Make the shower an exception rather than the rule.

Pamper yourself when you bathe. Use a bath oil, or a bubble bath, or an after-bath lotion, whichever you prefer. They all soften and subtly scent. Choose one in your favorite fragrance and use it lavishly. You can use an unscented mild soap, like Ivory, or a soap in the same perfume family as your bath oil. If it's not the same, it should at least be compatible, florals with florals, spice with spice, and so on.

We all have some problem areas that need special attention. You may have one or, happily, none at all. In any case, you might pay extra attention to these areas so that they won't become problems. Your back needs extra care, and you should have a cloth, sponge, or brush that will reach it. An excellent piece of bathing equipment is a loofah. This is a natural sponge which is dried to a special hardness and is marvelous for stirring up skin circulation. Use it for your knees and elbows, too.

Feet can so easily be ugly. They needn't be. After you step out of the tub, oil the cuticles of your toenails and push them back with an orange stick. Pumice off heel calluses with a lava stone or ease them off with a special lotion made for the purpose. "Pretty·Feet" is most effective, and you can use it for your hands as well. After your bath, dry your feet gently, especially between the toes, and fluff powder over them generously. Buff your toenails to a luster, unless you're planning on a pedicure. In that case, be sure to separate your toes with cotton pads before applying polish. This will keep the polish from smearing and wrecking the pedicure.

A generous fluff-on of your favorite dusting powder is a fitting finish to the whole bath routine. It gives you a feeling of luxury that can be the key to your whole day's attitude.

An Effective Deodorant

A deodorant that works is a must. Almost everyone today uses some kind of deodorant, but often it isn't as effective as another brand might be. You have to experiment until you get the right one for you. And even then, a product may work for you for years and then suddenly lose its potency, and you're in trouble. You must keep alert and be ready to switch, if necessary.

A certain amount of perspiration is natural and necessary, but a deodorant or an antiperspirant is standard equipment for any woman who wants to be dainty and feminine. An antiperspirant controls the amount of perspiration and lasts longer; a deodorant removes the odor but doesn't stop the perspiration, and has to be used more often. A model, of course, would have to use an antiperspirant, at least when she's working. Just think of the dresses that otherwise would be ruined. There are many good antiperspirants on the market, and the one you choose will be a matter of personal taste. Usually the liquids are best. As I say, you have to experiment. There are times when a girl can actually become immune to a certain product, and a change is the only answer.

I've discovered a method that I find works very well. The secret is to use an antiperspirant at night before you go to bed. I have spoken with a doctor about this and he says that if the body rests with an antiperspirant, the product will become more effective. Apparently when you apply it and then move around, it doesn't have a chance to do its work in closing the pores.

An antiperspirant is not harmful, but you have to exercise good judgment when using it. If it begins to irritate you, then stop using it. Of course, you never use it right after shaving. You could apply it before shaving, or a while after. Most of these products will last for a full day.

Keep Yourself Hair-Free

Your legs and underarms should be free of hair at all times. There are four methods of hair removal: shaving, depilatories, waxes, and electrolysis (permanent).

SHAVING. It has been said that when you shave, the hair grows back faster and longer. Not true. The cut ends may appear thicker as they grow out, but if you keep shaving regularly—as you must—it won't matter. It's about the quickest method, and you can choose between an electric shaver or a regular razor with a shaving cream or lotion.

USING DEPILATORIES. These are chemical formulas that go underneath the surface of your skin and lift the hair out. The results last longer, but so does the process. Also, you have to be careful to test for allergies before using. Some girls are completely allergic to most of these chemicals and will have to avoid them. There is a chance that one particular depilatory may be right, but this isn't a thing I'd advise you to experiment with. There are special formulas for removing facial hair or leg hair, and there is one product that is said to work well with either.

WAXING. A wax treatment is generally the most effective, as it will keep your skin free from hair for a period of four to six weeks. On the other hand, the process takes longer and isn't too easy to handle. It can be done professionally or you can do it yourself. The method: A wax is usually heated (some can be used cold, but aren't as efficient), smoothed on, allowed to cool, and finally stripped off. As it comes off, it takes the hair with it.

ELECTROLYSIS. This involves the use of an electric needle, and a highly skilled technician. It should *always* be done by an expert, and is definitely not a project for do-it-yourselfers. It is a delicate, difficult, and expensive process. The advantages are enormous, though, as this type of hair removal is permanent. Be sure that you select a technician who knows what she or he is doing. Hair has been known to grow back after some electrolysis removals, but circumstances have been unique in each case. Generally, results are permanent.

Note: Shaving is best for legs and underarms, waxing for legs and face, and depilatories for either.

LIGHTENING FACIAL HAIR

You can lighten facial hair instead of removing it. We prefer that you use this method. You can buy various brands of bleaching cream or make your own. Usually you don't leave any bleach on longer than five minutes. Remove it gently with a washcloth and warm water. If your hair still isn't as light as you want it, bleach again in a day or two. You also can bleach the hair on your arms and upper thighs. You never shave these areas—just bleach—but you do shave from ankle to knee.

For Beautiful Hands

For a model, beautiful hands can be more than just part of an overall beauty picture. They can lead to extra jobs as a hand model and, of course, will be an asset in getting any type of assignment. The way to genuinely beautiful hands is constant care.

A hand lotion or cream is as necessary to you as any item in your equipment. Frequent washing removes oils, wind roughens hands, cold-weather chapping can crack or tear the skin and cause hangnails. A lotion or cream prevents this by restoring moisture and oils after they're gone and, if you use it before exposure to the elements, it will actively reduce the rate of moisture evaporation.

Use your hand lotion after you wash your hands, after any kind of housework (if you do any), before you go out into the cold and after you come back from it, and before you go to bed at night. There are so many excellent preparations available that you won't have any trouble finding a good one. Another trick I like, and find most effective, is to smooth hands with Vaseline and cover them with soft gloves before going to bed. This will keep your skin soft and smooth, and work wonders with hangnails, if you have any.

A good idea is to keep some of your favorite hand preparation handy wherever you're likely to be—in the kitchen, bedroom, bathroom, and don't forget to put some in your model's hatbox. It can become second nature to smooth on a drop or two whenever you think you need it.

Don't forget that your arms and particularly your elbows need cream or lotion almost as much as your hands. Elbows have a tendency to get rough if neglected, so use the lotion regularly, and rub your elbows occasionally with lemon juice.

THE PERFECT MANICURE

Your nails are part of the picture when you're working on lovely hands. So big a part, in fact, that just one broken nail can spoil the whole effect, even though your hands are smooth and the other nine nails are perfect. You should work hard on having nice nails—and this means two manicures a week, which you can do at home—and using cuticle cream or Vaseline at night.

Naturally, you'll occasionally have manicures done at a beauty salon. It's such a luxurious feeling to just sit back and have everything done for you—hair, nails, the works!—but there isn't always time, and two manicures a week can turn into quite an expensive item. It's easy to learn to do your own nails. You'll need an easy method to follow and the proper equipment:

Warm soapy water (a mild liquid detergent will do)
Rinse water
Soft towel
Cuticle clippers
Hand cream or lotion
Nail file and emery boards
Orange stick

Polish
Polish remover and cotton pads
Nail buffer

First, remove your old polish with the remover and cotton pads. Remover-soaked pads are available in cosmetic departments, but I think these are best reserved for emergencies. When you have plenty of time, you can use cotton and remover, which cost much less proportionately. File the nails in one direction with a fine emery board. Avoid sharp points; the oval shape is the best. Dip the fingers in soapy water, rinse, and dry.

Now apply hand cream around your nails. This will soften dry skin and make it easier to clear away dead cuticle. Apply cuticle remover and push cuticle back with orange stick. Dip the fingers in soapy water again, soak for a few minutes, and dry. Clip off hangnails and rough cuticle with clippers. You'll have to practice this until you get the knack, but don't ever use nail scissors. Rinse your hands in clear water, dry them. Now you can finish shaping your nails. If any nails have been broken, file the rest of them down to as near the same length as possible. If all but one nail are perfect, just file the broken one and apply a false nail. I'll show you how to do this later.

Next, go around each nail with a cotton-tipped orange stick that has been dipped in oil, then buff each nail briskly. Now you're ready for your polish.

Your nail polish will last longer if you use a base coat and an overcoat in addition to the color. Slick the base coat on first, polish next (one or two coats), and then the overcoat. You can prevent premature chipping if you make sure that each coat of polish dries thoroughly before you apply the next one. This goes for base coat and overcoat, too.

ART OF APPLYING FALSE NAILS

When an ordinary girl breaks a nail, her best bet is to file the rest down to match, apply colorless or pale pearl polish, and wait for all nails to grow in again. When a model breaks a nail, there's no such easy way out for her. She'll have to apply a false nail, sometimes ten false nails. This is the easiest way to do it:

Try on your nails for size before you begin. If they need shortening, it is wiser to trim them from the base rather than from the tip. There are artificial nails for every shape of natural nail. The soft, neutral colors are best. If they need flattening or bending so that they'll conform to your own, you can dip them in hot water and shape them to suit. These are pretty fair nails and I find they hold well.

The major trick is to be sure to give yourself a good manicure before (omitting the polish, of course), and when you put the glue on, be sure to put it on both the real and the false nails. Have your false nails all lined up—all ten ready to put on—and have the glue on them and on your own. Let the glue get tacky. About two or three minutes is plenty, but you'll be able to tell because the glue starts to bubble. Press the false nail into place, push it close to the cuticle, down by the half-moon, press, and hold. Do all five nails on one hand before progressing to the other.

That's all. You're through. You can go off with fabulous nails, and it makes such a difference in your hands.

I do not recommend, though, that a girl wear false nails all the time. A rather strange thing can happen if you do. We've experienced this with our own models—including myself—who tried wearing them all the time. Within about six months in my case—less for others, depending on the structure of the individual nail—the glue begins to pit the real nails. If you wear them constantly, this is what will happen. The glue starts tearing and shredding the outer layer of your nail; the top layer starts peeling off and becomes tissue thin, a decidedly unhealthy condition.

I would say, then, that wearing false nails is not good as a steady thing but it's ideal for assignments. Once you have the feel of it, it doesn't take long to take them off or put them on again if you have them ready. Read the directions carefully.

Let Your Eyes and Your Smile Sparkle

There's more to facial beauty than faultless features and a cool hand with makeup. If your eyes don't sparkle and your teeth don't glow, forget about being a model! I'm going into inner motivation for this in my chapter on personality but, for purely physical aspects, there are a few things you ought to check on, and they definitely come under grooming and basic care.

It would be almost superfluous to say anything about keeping your teeth clean. You wouldn't have gotten this far on your way to a modeling career if you didn't know your teeth have to be shining and clean. If they are hard to whiten, there are harmless tooth cosmetics that will do the trick and, as I mentioned in a previous chapter, if there are minor imperfections it would pay you to have your orthodontist correct them. Of course, keep a tiny, portable breath purifier in your bag at all times.

A girl may be an expert with her eye makeup, but she'll be wasting her time if she doesn't pay some attention to the physical well-being of her eyes. Besides the necessity of good vision for any line of work, you should know that healthy eyes are beautiful eyes. If you're squinting and straining to see, you won't look your best at any time, and you'll be carving out wrinkles that will catch up with you in the not too distant future!

You may need glasses. If they're for reading only, they won't interfere with your modeling. If you're so nearsighted that you need glasses all the time, you'd better inquire about contact lenses. Not everyone can wear them comfortably, but if you're one of those who can, you have a built-in benefit right there. You can change your eye color as easily as you change your eye makeup color.

If you have any vision problems at all, visit your optometrist right away. If your vision is perfect, or near perfect, have your eyes examined at least once a year anyway.

Be sure to have the proper lighting conditions when you're doing any kind of work at home. Soft-focus light is best. Bright lights are dangerous, if you look directly into them. Those of you who plan to do fashion photography, especially, will be working with very bright lights. It seems hardly necessary to remind you not to look directly into them but, just in case, don't! By the same token, don't look directly at the sun unless you're wearing dark glasses.

Give your eyes a rest once in a while. If you're doing close work, take time off to glance across the room or out of a window for a second. Then close your eyes for a count of thirty.

It's best not to work your eyes too hard, but sometimes you must and there's no way out of it. Keep a good brand of medically formulated eyedrops on hand for quick, though temporary, relief. For longer lasting relief, and if you have enough time, soak cotton pads in witch hazel, then gently press the pads over your eyes, and lie down for about ten to fifteen minutes. Keep the witch hazel in the refrigerator, and the cool pads will feel wonderful.

Always keep an eyewash solution on hand for rinsing out dirt and grime that will find its way into your eyes in spite of the protective reflexes of your eyelids. You can either make your own solution, with boric acid and water according to directions, or buy any of the excellent formulas on the market.

One last hint concerning the tender, loving care your eyes deserve. Always keep a small bottle of your favorite eyedrops with you, in your purse and in your model's kit. It may turn out to be just the pickup you'll need on a busy, tiring day.

WARDROBE AND FITTINGS

A Model's Basic Wardrobe

Certain items must be part of a model's basic, permanent wardrobe. You must have lingerie and accessories you can use on assignments, and it's a good idea to save these things only for assignments. Then you won't be caught short when you have to go out on a job.

Start out with one of everything. You can always add extras to your original list. You will need girdles, bras, slips, hosiery, shoes, gloves, scarves, and jewelry. Other, or special, accessories will usually be provided by the dress shop or salon.

BASIC LIST

GLOVES
One pair of each:
Short black kid, plain
Short taupe kid, plain
Short beige kid, plain
Ten-button beige kid, plain
Opera-length white nylon stretch

Two pairs: short white nylon

Extras: sport gloves, knits, cutouts, different colors,
          opera-length black nylon stretch

The three pairs of short gloves are in the three neutrals that will go with anything. In the ten-button length, your beige will suffice; beige goes with so many things. If your costume has a three-quarter sleeve, and you want your glove to come up to it, this will be a pretty safe glove to have. Start out with one pair of opera-length stretch nylon evening gloves, but I'd like to see a girl have two pairs if she's going out professionally, so get your black ones next. Always have two pairs of short white nylon, and wash them after each wearing.

The more work you have, the more your glove wardrobe grows. As you add extras, you can get the bulky ones, the cut-outs, and the knits, as well as indulging yourself in various key colors. All your gloves must be in excellent condition and absolutely spotless. Print your initials inside each pair.

SCARVES (squares and long shapes)
Red
Yellow
Green

Blue
Black and white polka dot or stripe
Extras

Any color that looks well on you. Prints that are classic in pattern.

At the moment, scarves are very big news in accessories. They can be worn different ways around the neck and head. Look in the fashion magazines and copy the ideas you find there. Soft silk is seen more frequently; however, chiffon is most adaptable inside a suit neckline and will lie gracefully. Should you be modeling for a dress shop that does not carry scarves, by having your own scarves you will be ready to add one that will enhance the garment you are modeling.

Save the cardboard rollers from your paper towels, or something of the sort, and use them for packing your scarves. You only have to make one fold in the middle of your scarf—two at the most—and wind it around your roller. Put a little pin in it to keep it taut, then pack all these rolls in a plastic bag. It's a convenient way to carry them and keeps all your scarves wrinkle-free.

You'll be prepared if you have a red, a green, and a blue scarf. Select the colors that are most flattering to your skin tones.

HOSIERY
Two pairs of natural beige panty hose or body stockings
Two pairs of black sheer panty hose (bikini-type top or nude)

Today's model will have a variety of hose to use for evening, sports, and daytime fashions. The fashion coordinator or designer will let you know what type she wants to show with the clothes. Be prepared and always have two pairs of the same color in the sheer type. If your panty hose are too long, your girdle can be used to hold them up taut. With the very short styles you will sometimes have to remove your girdle and wear only the panty hose. Remember, if you are up on a runway the audience can sometimes see under your dress, and girdles are not pleasing to look at when you make a turn. You can wear bikini panties under panty hose if you have a completely nude shade.

GIRDLES
One white panty girdle
One black panty girdle
One model's white roll-on girdle

The white roll-on takes inches off. It's a straight tubular girdle and you can roll it on and take as much as 3 inches from your hips, depending on where you do the squeezing!

BRAS
One white natural-fit bra
One black natural-fit bra

One white padded bra or padding to add (padding described below)
One white low-back strapless ("Merry Widow" type)
One black low-back strapless ("Merry Widow" type)
One waist cincher

Your bras should have a natural fit, to give a very soft look. As a rule, a model does not need stays or padding. She should have padding available for one bra, if a dress calls for it. Be certain that your bras fit well and give a natural look to the bust line.

SLIPS

One fitted white nylon taffeta slip that zips
One fitted black nylon taffeta slip that zips
One white full slip, plain
One black full slip, plain

Taffeta is best because it repels static electricity and keeps your clothes from clinging to you. Half-slips should zip and be closely fitted so that there won't be any bulk or bulges underneath your clothes.

It might be a good idea to include a pretty camisole top. You might have to wear a sheer blouse, in which case your bra should not show through.

SHOES

One pair of each (All pumps with closed heel and toe)

Fall – Winter

Black kid pumps, plain
Various bows and buckles, to change the look
Taupe pumps, plain
Taupe boots
White and black silk evening

Extras:

One pair of red pumps
Whatever colors you want in your wardrobe

Spring – Summer

Black patent pumps, plain
White leather
Beige leather
White or natural sandals
Sandals in any "in" color for the season; no thongs
Use same evening shoes, as for fall and winter

Extras:

One pair of red shoes
Whatever other colors you want in your wardrobe

All of your shoes should fit beautifully. They should not slip off your heels, and should cling to your feet like gloves. You'll need plain black pumps, and you might invest in a few smart sets of bows or buckles to change the look occasionally. Next comes a pair of taupe pumps. Taupe is that very soft, leathery brownish hue that goes so well with blacks, browns, and many different colors.

It seems as if boots are here to stay, so by all means have a pair of fashionable boots in a color that you can wear with everything. Taupe would be good, as would beige or bone. For evening, you can usually get by with black and white evening shoes in silk, peau de soie, or faille. Keep them very carefully, just for shows.

I think that the very first pair of extra shoes a girl should buy would be red. It's a color that is great with navy or any of shade of blue you might be wearing. After the red, you could get whatever colors you might want that prevail in your wardrobe.

Your basic spring-summer shoes would include black patent-leather pumps. These are not restricted to spring and summer but it would be up to the designer to decide if he wants a patent-leather look in winter. There is some controversy on this among designers, but patent is more acceptable for spring and summer wear. Your beige leather and white leather shoes should be plain, basic pumps with the heels and toes intact. No slings and no cutout toes. Sandals for summer, of course, in white or natural, unless there's something very new that season such as gold. Your extras can be red again, or any other color that might be worn well with your other things.

All of your shoes must be good-looking, new heel and toe shapes, in good taste, and *always* in good repair.

JEWELRY

One short pearl necklace, one or two strands
Pearl earrings to match
One long pearl necklace, one or two strands
Long rhinestone evening earrings
One gold chain
One basic gold pin
One silver chain
One basic silver pin
Gold earrings
Silver earrings

You'll use your own jewelry only when you model for a store that doesn't supply it. You should have some standard items in your wardrobe. Pearls, gold, and silver amply cover your ordinary needs. One pearl necklace should be short and fit around a jewel neckline. It can either be one- or two-strand, and you'll need simple pearl earrings to go with this. A longer strand of pearls—matinee or opera length—

is good to have, too, and you can wear it with the same pearl earrings.

For evening costumes, long rhinestone earrings will be perfect. Maybe you can add long pearl ones too, so that you have a choice.

Have a gold and a silver pin. Either adds a basic touch to a very simple dress. You'll need gold and silver earrings—a pair of each—to go with these accents. Keep them simple; the button kind is best. If your hairdo or a hat would hide them, it won't be necessary for you to wear earrings at all. Gold and silver chains will be good for sportswear.

If you ever work for a large department store, you will usually receive all the accessories you'll need from the respective departments. Then you won't need all of these things, but our models here, and in other communities, supply their own because they work for shops which do not carry accessories. They learn to add the proper accessories to the costumes they're showing, so that they're not just walking out with a dress that isn't properly accessorized.

Wherever you are, you should have all your accessories in your wardrobe, and with you on every job, so that you'll never be caught short on an assignment. The model who is always ready and on time with everything she needs is the model that the shop or the photographer will remember and call for again.

A Warning. Do not take expensive jewelry with you on an assignment, or any amount of money larger than you will need for fare or food. The reason: You are never sure about dressing-room conditions, and why tempt anyone interested in your extra cash? Be wise, don't make it available.

Fittings

When you are asked to go out on a fitting, there are certain necessary items that you must take along. Generally, you would take a tote bag containing the things you'll need. You should have a head covering, different types of shoes, various types of bras, and you should be prepared to adjust to different sizes with a model's girdle. You'll find the ways to do this in the following section.

Assuming that you have everything you need with you, you will walk into the shop, introduce yourself, and ask for the fashion coordinator. You will be directed to a dressing room. Undress and, as the clothes you are to wear are handed to you, get into them quickly. Step out, walk away from the coordinator with real confidence, and do a turn to show how the garment looks on you. It may be decided right then and there whether the costume is acceptable for the show.

Remove the dress and hang it on a hanger. Sometimes a salesgirl will take care of all the preliminaries such as pinning, buttoning, and adjusting. If not, you take care of this later.

Put on the second garment, step out, and do a model's turn. Watch and observe the coordinator's expression. You'll know whether another turn is necessary. Perhaps you'll just do a quick walkaway, get the coordinator's approval, and that's it. You'll have to learn to interpret expressions.

To be quick and efficient at fittings is vital. Work with the clothes a little bit, too, so that the coordinator will see you're comfortable handling them. Get them to look right and feel right on your body before you take one step out of the dressing room.

You have no idea how many models merely put on a garment and haven't put it on right. Shoulder seams aren't where they should be or the belt needs adjusting. This all takes practice, of course, but practice makes perfect.

This is why modeling is such a great experience for a girl. You do nothing but take clothes off and put them on all day long, and you work with designers who insist on details that will make the clothes look right.

Check carefully with your coordinator for each garment that is selected. What are you going to wear with it? Do you have the correct shoes in your personal wardrobe, or is the shop supplying them? If it's necessary to take a notebook and jot things down, do it. Know what you have to bring from your own wardrobe for each costume, and be clear about it. If you're to have six changes, know what shoes you'll need, what gloves. Will the store be supplying the basic accessories? Or do you bring your own? Jot all the information down. Then you'll be safe.

Be sure that you're neat and clean. Your underclothing should be impeccably clean, and not held together with pins, or torn. It does happen! No model should be perspiring. Never be seen going for a fitting with curlers in your hair or without makeup. How can they possibly judge how that costume is going to look if you look as if you've just got out of bed? Don't walk in for a fitting in slacks. Walk in looking every inch a model.

Sometimes you may even have to bring a prop from home. It's possible. If you'll be wearing a tennis outfit and the store can't supply it, ask them, "Would you like me to bring a tennis racquet to the fashion show?"

They'll be happy that you're concerned with showing the frock to its best advantage by using the right props, even if they don't take you up on it. Whether or not they do, your suggestion will certainly be appreciated.

I might add that dress shops sometimes forget about time. Actually, a fitting should not take more than an hour, often much less. A model need not be taken advantage of, spending three hours for a fitting while the store's personnel waits on customers. This is why it is so important to know the exact hour of your fitting, and that the shop even knows your size in advance so that the time consumed can be pared down.

True, customers are very important, but those in charge should not be discourteous to the model, either. This is why fitting time should be paid time. Unfortunately, this is not true in all cities. A good rate would be half the model's ordinary fee. At medium rates, the fee would include a fashion show. I would normally consider an hour sufficient for an average fitting. If the coordinator asks all the models to come at one time so that she can see certain things, it would take longer. However, if the sizes for the girls have been selected in advance, it can go rather quickly. Either way, you should be paid for this time.

Should you feel you're being taken advantage of, remember you must be a lady, even if you have been forgotten. Step out and say something like, "I'm terribly sorry, but my fitting time was at two o'clock and I did allow an hour and I have an appointment at three. Is it at all possible to hurry this along?"

Be nice about it. Tell those in charge that you have an appointment and you've allowed an hour. Don't sit back in the dressing room for half an hour without anyone helping you. Wait five minutes and then let them know. It's quite possible for them to get carried away in their business, too. The customer is still the one who's paying the rent, so let's not be impertinent or insistent or demanding. You can still be a lady and be gracious about informing them that you're waiting and may have been forgotten.

We'll just do a quick review of how to show your costume at a fitting. Get into the garment, step out of the dressing room, and walk away from the fashion coordinator, who is going to have to judge whether it's right on you and should be used for the showing.

Walk out, do a pivot, turn around, and smile. Get the feel of the dress, or suit, or whatever it is. Let the coordinator see a little of how you would handle it onstage. It isn't as if you were going to do a complete format. Just walk away and do a turn. Look at her face and, if she looks quizzical, do another turn to give her the opportunity to see if she wants to have this shown.

She'll probably say, "That's fine; that will do," or, "No, I don't like it." Take your cue from her expression, then go back to the dressing room, get into another outfit, and go through the whole thing again.

A MODEL'S BAG OF TRICKS

A model has to be ready for any type of emergency that may arise during an assignment. Ideally, the outfit she is to wear will fit her perfectly, her skin will be glowing and blemish-free, her hair will have bounce and body, and she'll never, *never* have a cold or feel in any way under the weather.

That's the way it should be and — I hope — the way it will be for you most of the time. But models are human, and so are designers, and photographers, and fashion coordinators, and things do go wrong occasionally. What do you do when a costume doesn't quite fit, or a blemish pops up, or you come down with a dilly of a cold on the day of the big job?

Well, for one thing, don't panic. There are any number of handy helpers you can keep in your "model's bag of tricks," and they can do anything from easing over a minor rough spot to turning a near disaster into a triumph. I've worked out many of these myself, while others are from the personal experience of some of our top models.

Some of these tricks lie in "surprise" accessories you actually can keep in your kit, and others are just ideas that you'll keep in your head. However you tote them along with you, I know that they'll be of inestimable help to you as you go along. You should be able to tackle the unforeseeable in almost every case if you're properly armed with your own special "bag of tricks."

Here are some of ours. As time goes on, you'll surely find or devise some new ones that work well for you. Add them to your list and, if you want to be really generous, pass them along.

Some of My Own

FOR A LARGER BUST SIZE. Sometimes you'll need to create the illusion of a larger bust size. Possibly the dress is cut for a fuller bust line and it won't look quite right unless you fill it up. Save your old hosiery (only the natural-colored nylons) and cut off the tops and feet. Have a larger-size bra in your wardrobe and stuff it with this hosiery.

This gives a soft, natural look. The hosiery is ideal for this because it's flesh-colored and soft. The bra that many of our girls are wearing now features the natural bust line. It's a sheer nylon bra that just rounds the contour and only needs a little extension.

Some models still use little foam bust pads or fillers. They're both used, but the softer, more natural line is what we want.

TO CREATE MORE ROUNDNESS TO THE BODY. If a girl has to fill out her rib cage, her waist, side or back of her hip, there are tricks to accomplish this. There are, of course, girdles that have pads already built in if a girl really is in need of this type of thing. You can round out and mold your own figure to fit a garment very quickly, though, without the use of a padded girdle.

Maybe you're wearing a size 8 in the first part of a fashion show and you're expected to get into a size 10 in another part. You'll have to adjust to this quickly. You'd have to have a larger waist, rib cage, and hips. There are two things you can do.

1. Using a regular longline girdle, you can stuff sanitary napkins under the girdle wherever you need the extra inches—around the waist, down the sides for a little more hip, down the back, in under the longline's bra to bring out the rib cage. It sounds like a strange remedy, I know, but you'd be surprised how this particular type of bulk will tend to fill out the clothes, making them fit and look much better.

2. Another idea that I like involves shredded rubber. Buy a big bag of shredded foam rubber. You can generally get this in the sewing section of a department store, or even, occasionally, in a hardware store. Now, take the old hosiery you've been saving, cut off the tops and feet, and stitch across the bottom. Stuff the stockings lightly with foam rubber, making sure to do this evenly, and stitch across the top.

Make several of these in various lengths and different sizes, four inches to eight inches, even ten, and longer ones to go halfway around the waist or even completely around the waist. This would be up to you. You'd have to know what you need occasionally, but you must have different lengths to be adequately equipped. These foam-filled stockings are very soft, and you can push them around a lot more than the sanitary napkins. I know models who use both. I personally prefer the rubber ones, but the napkins are handy. A model should carry these in her hatbox at all times.

FOR FLEXIBILITY. A good model should be flexible. You may get an assignment because you're a size 8 and able to wear a size 10. You should be able to wear at least two different sizes. Some models can wear almost three different sizes, but this depends on the manufacturer and how he cuts his clothes. With the stuffed stockings or napkins, and the proper girdle, you can easily go from one size to the next and back.

The proper foundation is important. A model's girdle is essential for the girl who wants to be able to wear every type of costume in a fashion show. Familiarize yourself with the girdle and bra picture by going into a good department store, and look at the girdles the models wear.

TO WEAR A SMALLER SIZE. You can actually make your hips two inches smaller with a model's girdle, if it's necessary. You have to roll it down, as you would hosiery, and slip it up on your waist. It is constructed as a tubular girdle and when you roll it down your body, it is so tight that you can squeeze in your hips and be able to wear a whole size smaller. For some of those long, slim formals that demand narrow hips, you may need to come down one size.

Makeup and Miscellaneous

QUICK BLOTTER FOR AN OILY COMPLEXION. A fast repair for an oily complexion makes use of a bit of special tissue and a pressed powder compact. When the shine comes through your foundation, and this is easy enough under studio lights, blot your face with one of the specially treated linen tissues made just for this purpose, then pat on a film of pressed powder for a smooth matte finish. The treated tissues remove the oil without disturbing your existing makeup. Pat or blot, though, don't rub. Carry these tissues with you at all times. Another good thing to have, if your skin tends to be oily, is any one of the marvelously efficient blotter-pressed powders now on the market. These products really blot out oils as they smooth a fresh finish over your face.

CHANGE YOUR LIPSTICK COLOR IN A JIFFY. If the lipstick you're wearing is too red or orange for the costume you're showing, you can cool the color with an overlay of a blue-toned lip gloss. On the other hand, if your lipstick is too rosy or blue-toned, you can warm it up with a gold-toned gloss. If you just want a lighter tint of the shade you're wearing, a white pearl gloss will do the trick. Never travel to any job without these three do-everything lip glosses.

TO MAKE A FRENCH TWIST IN A HURRY. You may have an assignment that calls for a quick hairstyle change, with the choice left up to you. A French twist will often answer the purpose. The simplest way to make one: Brush your hair to the highest point on the crown where the twist is to end. Grasp the ends in one hand as if you were going to make a ponytail, and deftly make one full twist. Secure the ends temporarily but firmly, which will manage the bulk and still leave your hands free to make a neat job of the actual twist from the nape line up. Keep your hairpins well hidden, locking each one into the next. Final step, tuck all the exposed ends neatly underneath.

SPEEDY SET FOR SHORT-NOTICE ASSIGNMENTS. If you get a hurry-up call and your coiffure is limp, and all your hairpieces are at the hairdresser (heaven forbid!), you can liven up your set in less than half an hour. Needless to say, this should never happen; you should always have some type of hairpiece at hand. Just in case, barely dampen your hair with water and wind it on rollers across the top section. Pin the ends in big, open curls and spray lightly with your holding spray. (Cologne is good, too.) Set this way, most hair dries in less than a half hour. When dry, brush out briskly, and finger it into place.

REPAIRING NAIL POLISH. This isn't really a repair, it's a redo. Take off the chipped or damaged polish with a polish-remover pad (much quicker and more convenient than cotton and remover), and let the nail dry for a second. Slick on the fresh polish quickly and evenly in just three strokes, one in the middle and one on either side, overlapping the middle stroke. Wave your hands in the air for speedy drying. This won't last long, but it's great when you're in a rush.

10

A MODEL'S RESPONSIBILITIES

There isn't a girl who has studied modeling who hasn't developed more of a personality, more confidence, more grace and charm. There is an inner feeling that comes with this. There are responsibilities that come with it, too. The very fact that you are a model must keep you extremely aware of how you act at all times. People look at you—with admiration or envy, as the case may be—so it's up to you to set the proper note.

You are looked upon as a leader. You must be a leader. Keep abreast of new fashions in makeup, hairstyling, and the ways of wearing accessories. Be quick to change. Remember, fashion presents a hectic milieu. By its very nature, it is based on change. You have to be able to change with it. Trends alter every six months. Experiment with what is new. Not always drastically, but just enough to keep you that extra little bit ahead. Keep your eyes open. Learn to adapt and change.

Responsibility also lies in developing your personality. Practice to improve yourself constantly, and to be a model at all times when you're out in public. Be well groomed, impeccably dressed, well-mannered, and soft-spoken.

Be perfect for your public, and let your agency help you in every way. Every top model should be with an agency.

AGENCY OR FREE-LANCE?

I can't imagine any girl wanting to be on her own, unless there isn't an agency in her town, which I'll go into later. If you are qualified and an agency will accept you, there is absolutely no reason to try to free-lance. There are exceptions, of course. Models like Jean Shrimpton or Twiggy have their own personal managers.

There are advantages in being with a good agency. It's your protection. Above all, I think, is the prestige that a good agency can give you. You must recognize the fact that no one knows you as yet. You would have to advertise and spend money on the overhead of a business. You'd need a secretary, and a telephone service, and you'd have to take space in the Yellow Pages, all so that people would know where you are at any given time. You would continually have to make the rounds, which can be very trying, as well as making you unavailable for jobs that might come in while you are so engaged.

WHAT YOUR AGENCY DOES FOR YOU

1. Has a business office open to show and sell your talents.
2. Provides contacts for you.
3. Manages your complete schedule.
4. Bills your clients and handles your collections.
5. Acts as a complete business telephone service for you.
6. Protects you by checking out clients who wish to hire you.
7. In most cases, gets a rate of remuneration for your services that you would not get as an individual.

8. Mails out a vast amount of pictures, letters, and literature to potential customers.
9. Sells your talents better than you can sell yourself.

You'll still have to make the rounds in any city for your agency, because it is part of your job, but it will be organized. If you sign with a good agency, you will be better off. It lends you prestige, and you will have much more exposure. You work with your agency and cooperate with it.

If you don't get assignments, you might possibly change your appearance a little, to see if it could make a difference. Keep your pictures updated. Do everything your agency desires of you, and *keep in touch with it constantly*. Don't sit complacently at home and say, "They'll call me."

You have to keep in touch with your agency and find out what you must do to possibly obtain more assignments. They want to work with you also, and each area and its needs would be different. An agency in a small city is not going to expect as much, but at least it would have something to offer clients when they call. Being loyal to your agency is important.

I don't know of a top model who hasn't been with an agency. You must sign exclusively with your agency. This is important to a client looking for a particular type of model, and he will be assured of seeing new faces when he walks into each agency.

You must remember the agency is working for you every day, through the photos it shows, the use of studio facilities, and the tremendous amount of mail that is sent out on your behalf. If you did it yourself, you'd be sitting at the typewriter all day just working on your mail!

A girl who free-lances will find it isn't going to pay in the long run. For the few cents on the dollar you pay your agency — 10 percent or 15 percent, determined by the state you live in — it's like having a personal secretary. Actually, it is a personal secretary, and a business manager, and a publicist! It's well worth it because, after all, you don't pay it unless you earn it. And, believe me, the agencies have to pay their upkeep whether they have a job coming or not, so you're the one who's ahead of the game.

Read your model's contract thoroughly and understand it. If you decide to terminate the contract so that you can free-lance or go to another agency, know what you are doing, and handle details in a businesslike manner. If you're in doubt about your responsibilities, have an attorney read the contract through carefully and get his advice. Most contracts are legal and must be carried out as agreed. On an average, contracts can bind you from thirty days to two years.

When considering making a change, check out the new agency with models already in their employ. In this way you can find out about its policies, and whether it is reliable and reputable.

So sign up with a good, reputable agency. Always carry your agency cards and picture composites with you when you're contacting dress shops, photographers, and any of your "go-see" calls. Leave your composites and your agency's phone number. In making contacts, always give your agency's phone number.

Always look professional, and always be neat.

If you live and intend to work in a city which has no agency at all, you necessarily will have to free-lance. If there are only a few dress shops and only so much modeling available, you will have to make potential clients aware of your qualifications.

Go to the shops and leave something with them such as pictures, a personal card, or a mimeographed sheet listing your credits and experience. You must keep your photographs current so that the people you're working for will see you as you are and be able to judge whether they can use you.

You might have a composite made up. You'll see sample headsheets and composites in Chapter 13. It is a wise investment to have glossy photos made, but try to choose a good photographer who will capture the essence of you. Try to show three different expressions. A good portfolio of photographs will be an asset if you decide to leave your city and apply to another agency.

How to Apply

If you're refused by several agencies, due to lack of training, what do you do then? Then you go to a good school and find out exactly what is wrong. They will usually be honest with you, though I think this is hard for a girl to accept.

In my own experience, I have had girls walk into my agency who say they've had training. I believe them. Either it was inadequate training, or maybe they just trained with a personal friend, but they were *not* models. This is so important.

You should walk in looking like a model. Have a new-fashioned look. Know how to do things that are in this book. It proves you are a model.

You can't fool an agency. Ask for an honest opinion. "Am I a type that you could use?" Be brave enough to accept what they say. When I tell a girl she needs training, I'm sincere about it. She really does need it.

Be willing to invest in your profession if you need training. Study and learn from this book, or pay an expert to help and guide you. Some people need another person's analysis to let them know what they need. If you don't believe the first person you ask, go to someone else and ask for an honest opinion. Ask three different sources who are known to be experts.

It's the same as consulting a doctor. If you want to know what's wrong with you and don't believe one doctor, you go to another, and you finally get the right diagnosis. So it is with modeling.

If I tell a girl she needs makeup, she needs it. If she doesn't know how to apply it, she can learn. If you don't know how to do all the various stage and runway formats, how to conduct yourself as a model and do the turns, you can learn them. Smooth them out and become a professional.

You would be surprised at the way girls have walked into agencies, and claimed to be professional models! A girl will walk in with over-bleached hair, an evening hairstyle in the daytime, have on far too much makeup, and not a new makeup. She will walk in with spike heels, no hosiery, ill-kept clothes, and say she's a fashion model! You wonder where she gets the nerve to do this, but she does! Because she may have been in one fashion show five years ago, or three, or even two years ago, doesn't make her the top model she would like to be.

Because you can do a basic Model's Pivot doesn't mean you're a full-fledged model. You must learn how to model effortlessly and do things right. You may have a natural grace, and still not know how to handle a coat onstage. You may be able to walk beautifully and maybe do a Model's Pivot, but you don't know how to work a stage or how to exit and enter. These are things that need to be refined.

Here, again, is where this book will be such a help to you. You may have had enough basic training so that you can come through and really learn it in this book, but then you go on to the next person and ask, "What's wrong with it? Tell me. What do I need?" When you can accept this, you're on your way.

Interviews — "Go-See" Calls

Part of a model agency's job is to set up your daily schedule of definite bookings and "go-see" calls and make sure that you know about them in advance. At the end of each day, you will either be given a typed schedule or a set of slips giving the information on your bookings. Sometimes you'll be notified by telephone.

These interviews are tremendously important. You are, in effect, selling *yourself*, so make sure that what clients see is thoroughly pleasing. First and foremost, you should be at your most appealing best. You must look like a model when you go to an interview. Have that real bandbox look, and be very much up-to-date for your particular city and area. Speak to the fashion coordinator or manager of the shop, or the photographer, or whomever you're scheduled to see.

Walk in as if you're very happy. Make it a rigid rule to be a least *a few minutes* early. I think about fifteen minutes early is a good idea. It's far better for you to wait than the client.

Find excuses to go back. If you don't get a job, don't ever be discouraged. Strangely enough, you may look entirely different to the same person if you wear a different color, hairstyle, or makeup. Psychologically, you never know why you are selected. You may be wearing a particular color. It could be your client's favorite color and he will, unconsciously, select you because he is drawn to it. It could be anything at all, besides your being the size needed.

After people get to know you a little more, they'll be more apt to call you. Your face registers with them. They'll remember you when they want a model, if they've seen you enough times.

So make sure they do see you often enough! Make excuses to remind them of you. Drop in to see their new styles, or stop in a minute just to say "Hello." Make an excuse that's plausible and make a point of going back regularly, especially when you know it's time for them to be thinking about getting ready for showings. Don't make a pest of yourself. Be tactful and casual, but see to it that they remember you and think of you favorably.

Don't forget to leave your agency card and your composites. Follow your agency's advice and you will not go wrong.

HOW TO CONDUCT YOURSELF

As a model, you are sure to be the center of attraction, offstage as well as on. Your own common sense and what you'll learn about developing your personality will help you in your private life, but there are certain things that are expected of you in your professional life. Your conduct at fittings, at fashion shows, how prepared you are for any eventuality. If you learn these things, clients will learn to look for you, and more jobs will be available.

Fittings

Be on time for your fittings. Check in with your coordinator immediately. Never put on a garment without covering your head with a cap or scarf. You should never allow anything to go over your head unless it's covered. If the dress has such a wide zipper opening that it's obvious you won't touch anything, then it doesn't matter. It is best, though, to be safe.

I think the little nylon caps that zip would be best, but here's a trick you can do with a scarf. Take a see-through chiffon scarf and put it over your head completely, with two points in front and two at the back. Take the two points at the back, bring them around in front and tie them in a knot under your chin. That will draw in the scarf so it holds your hair in place and keeps your makeup from smearing the clothes.

Wear a girdle, stockings, and take along a strapless bra. Check beforehand to see what particular clothes are needed, if you're modeling immediately after fittings. Of course, your underwear is clean, new-looking, never torn or pinned.

When you've stepped into the garment in the dressing room, step out of the dressing room, if there's space, and walk away from the coordinator. Walk out, do a graceful pivot, turn around, and smile. Don't do a whole format, but give the coordinator a chance to see how you would handle the costume onstage.

Never express your opinion, unless it's asked for. They know what they wish to show. Never throw the clothes around carelessly. Hang them on hangers when you have finished with them, unless there is someone there to assist you.

Never sit down, or lean against anything, with the costumes on. Don't smoke, drink, or eat while wearing them.

Always be helpful. Be efficient, friendly, and cooperative. Above all, a model must never be known as temperamental.

Fashion Show Time

Be on time. Report in and check the lineup sheet. Check your clothes and accessories. Unzip, unbutton, untie, or unsnap whatever garment needs it. (Your wardrobe assistant will probably have this done, but check it.) Have everything ready to step into. Have your shoes, accessories, and jewelry lined up and ready to wear.

If anything should be wrong with the clothing, report it immediately. Don't hesitate to ask for assistance from the wardrobe woman. When putting on the costumes, follow all of the above rules for fittings. Check your appearance and entrance picture in the mirror.

Practice backstage, if you have to, so that you can get the feel of the costume. You should be waiting to go onstage when the model you follow is already on.

When the show is ended, put your clothes and your accessories in order. Snap, button, zip, or tie the garments and put them back on the hangers. Check out with the coordinator and thank the wardrobe woman.

Be pleasant, modest, and poised. Don't be loud or boisterous, and never leave without permission. Always thank the people involved with the show.

What to Keep in Your Model's Hatbox

Actually, hardly any model ever carries a hatbox anymore. It's more likely to be a tote bag, but it's still usually called a hatbox in model's training.

As I mentioned when discussing your bag of tricks, a model must be prepared for any eventuality. This is why your hatbox should include anything you're apt to need. You should have:

1. A scarf or hood for your head. Possibly arm shields, though you shouldn't perspire if you're using the right antiperspirant.

2. Pins, clear nail polish, flesh-colored bandaids.

3. Several pairs of extra hosiery. *This is a must.*

4. A complete set of extra makeup; lipstick changes, or a yellow-toned and a blue-toned gloss to change the color of the lipstick you're wearing.

5. A jewelry box, gloves, scarves.

6. A selection of hairpieces. Probably carried in own box.

7. Correct lingerie.

8. Correct shoes.

Always check to see that your shoes are in A-1 condition, clean and well polished. Check with your coordinator regarding accessories, and add whatever is needed to your supplies.

This is a general outline of what your hatbox should contain. Exactly what kind of lingerie and accessories you should include is covered thoroughly in Chapter 9.

FASHION SHOW ETIQUETTE

Be proud to represent your agency. Everything you do will reflect on it.

Listen to the narrator.

Remember, you are modeling and selling clothes. If you have an accident, carry on gracefully with a smile. You won't be the first —or the last!—to make a mistake or have something unusual happen onstage.

One of my own models, for instance, got into a bit of a spot during a fashion show and she instinctively did the right thing. It was one of those trick stages, with little brass rings here and there on the stage. The model caught her heel in one of the rings. What she learned at one of our classes helped her.

We ask our students, "What do you do in unusual circumstances?" The answer—in the case of a shoe—is that if anything should happen at any time, just step out of your shoe.

Our model remembered, stooped down, worked her heel out easily by hand, put the shoe aside, slipped her foot back into it, did a model's turn, smiled, and walked off. The applause was deafening because she did this so gracefully.

We also have furs slip off the shoulders accidentally. This can happen, especially if you're wearing gloves and you lose control of handling the fur. It shouldn't happen, but it does. The way to handle this is to pick up the fur nonchalantly, drape it over your shoulder, and off you go.

If you drop an earring or something really small that cannot be seen onstage, it wouldn't be necessary to stoop and pick it up. This can be done afterward. Forget it and go off the stage. Any unusual happening that would be noticeable onstage is annoying and disturbing to the audience. Always get out of it gracefully. Convey the expression, "Well, look what happened to me!" Smile as if it hadn't happened at all and go offstage.

In my first years of modeling, I ran into a circumstance of this sort. I was wearing the spike heels that were in vogue at the time. The shoes were backless, and I was wearing a lavish lace hostess gown. In gliding down the stairs, the dress dropped to the step and got caught in the heel. I don't know how, but it did. I wasn't aware of this, so when I took another step I ripped almost the entire hemline in the back! It was hanging in practically a separate piece.

You do feel horrible about a thing like this, but you see that it's done, and there's nothing you can do about it, so you simply keep modeling and go offstage. This is definitely a "show-must-go-on" kind of thing. You must develop this within you. My advice to all models when something like this happens is, "Smile, and carry on as if nothing had happened."

KEEP UP WITH FASHION

One of the most important responsibilities a model has, I think, is to keep up with every facet of her profession. Never stop learning. If effective new techniques come up, study them and use them.

Go to fashion shows. No matter how many shows you participate in yourself, attend others. One of the models may do something different and create a beautiful look and a stunning effect. This is how each new technique is developed, because some model did it and it looked well, or because some imaginative director dreamed it up. See as many fashion shows as you can squeeze into a busy schedule, and you may pick up a pointer that can make a marvelous difference in your style.

The lessons you learn in this book will be amplified by your seeing a professional go through the motions. On the other hand, you may see some old, seldom-used movements or antiquated pivots being done. Don't be confused and think, "Oh, they don't do that." That's not true at all. It's just that the model hasn't learned the new methods, and you do know them.

Just keep on attending fashion shows until you see the models doing the new things. It is worth the price of the ticket to check in on the top shows—if you are in the big cities or near them—and watch the models work.

Besides helping you with your techniques, seeing fashion shows will keep you abreast of the new styles. I've already mentioned that you must be aware of the latest in makeup and hairstyles, but I must remind you to keep up with the world of fashion as well. On the surface, this sounds like unnecessary advice, but you'd be surprised how easy it is to become absorbed in your own little world of modeling, and forget the picture as a whole. Of course, pay attention to your current fashion coordinator or photographer or whomever you're working with, but be aware of everything that is going on in the fashion field.

Learn about designers. Get to recognize their names and, at least to a certain extent, the identifying characteristics of their clothes. Read the fashion magazines—especially if you're planning to be a photographic model—and see what the trends are. Even more than the magazines, read the daily fashion columns in your local newspapers. If you can, subscribe to *Women's Wear Daily*, or get a single copy once in a while. Newspapers come out every day, so the fashion news will get to you sooner than through the magazines, though not in such gorgeous detail.

Read fashion, think fashion, practically breathe fashion. This is a world you're going to be part of, hopefully, for a long, long time. You owe it to yourself—and to the clothes you model—to have as much knowledge about fashion and design as you have about modeling techniques.

The clothes you are showing are beautiful. You love them, not only because they are beautiful, but because you know what goes into their making, from the first glimmer in the designer's brain to the finished costumes so perfectly fitted on the models' figures.

Study. Learn. Be constantly ready for change—in a mode, in a trend, in a style. This is a model's responsibility—to the designers she serves and to the audience who looks to her as the last word in chic.

11

DEVELOPING YOUR PERSONALITY AND STYLE

CREATE AN INNER EMOTION

Modeling will develop your personality, but you must have a warm and outgoing feeling for the world around you. Learning the basic techniques of modeling and getting to know the feel of the clothes will help to round you out, but you must be friendly, have a natural love for beauty and life itself, and have a nature that knows the joy of giving. The art of showing clothes is the art of giving pleasure.

When you see a model working on a stage or a runway, how do you feel about her? What is your first impression when she makes her initial appearance onstage?

A model must create a theme for the clothes she's wearing. She must sell by making the audience love the look of that particular costume, and want to buy it! She has to make a woman see *herself* in that particular look. There is an inner emotion about clothes that must be felt if you are going to be an excellent model.

Let's pretend you are standing backstage, ready to model. Once you have the costume on, you must lose yourself completely to whatever the aim is in showing that particular garment and expressing the meaning of its style. Anyone reading this who has taken dramatic lessons will understand what I mean. Remember, to show true emotion, you must feel it with your mind as well as your body, your whole emotional self.

Does this sound silly? Not really. You must play-act to be possessed with a love for this particular costume. Never be passive about anything you're wearing. Develop a great imagination. I repeat:

Developing a great imagination makes a better model.

Let's imagine you are modeling a tailored pants suit and boots. Although you will know the stage routine you're planning to use with this, you should be able to do it without thinking. You'll know your hand positions, how your costume should be used to show details and lines, and now you must feel that pants suit.

How will you show it? Where are you walking in it? Not only on the stage. Put yourself into an emotional feeling about it. You're really walking in the country. So you walk briskly onto the stage with the same animated feeling you would have if you were walking in the country. Feel the sensations you would enjoy if you were doing this. It will show in your face and body. You will create an atmosphere to go with that particular suit. You must work with your body and mind together. You move in harmony with this.

I have seen girls do beautiful body formats, use their hands elegantly, but their faces show nothing. The audience doesn't get the feeling of that costume because the model has lost expression. You can learn, though, and improve by practicing and practicing. Use your imagination with this goal in mind, and have an artistic vision working with you.

Another good idea is to be always one step ahead of yourself mentally. When you know you're going over to a corner of a stage to do a turn, you do it mentally before you do it physically. You'll find that you'll do the actual turn more smoothly.

Example: Lift your hand — without thinking. Just lift it. Look in the mirror while you're doing this. Now, lift your hand again, but think about it first. Think of doing it smoothly. Mentally move the hand in the direction you plan to do it. Now *physically* lift your hand. Drop it, mentally. Now drop it, physically. Notice how much smoother the motion is.

Now, this may sound silly to you, but practice doing a turn physically. Now, mentally do that turn instead of just physically doing it, and it will come through more smoothly every time.

An actor must always be a step ahead of himself. You must be this in modeling as well.

Acting is an important part of modeling. You have to be an actress, even if in a fairly limited sense. Let's say, for instance, you're modeling something that's very high fashion, but that you think you look terrible in. You will look ridiculous if you don't know how to model it correctly.

Take the most bizarre high-fashion item you've seen lately, put it on the right model, and let her step out onstage with complete confidence. You don't have to like what you're modeling, but you have to be able to model it as if you do like it!

It can be quite amusing. I find that when we have some costume a model is wearing that she simply abhors—her distaste for it is so great—she will throw in her real acting ability and, because of her tremendous effort to like the garment, she shows it superbly. In many cases, she portrays it so well that she does much better with this than with the things she really likes, because she takes those so matter-of-factly.

It's happened many, many times where models have disliked a costume but, because they know they must bring every ounce of effort into it, they sell it. That's why we will always need *live* models, to let others get the same feeling of fun, and that perhaps the garment would be just right for the woman who buys it.

As an actress onstage, you must always be aware of what your next move will be, and I think anything in theatre can be used in modeling. Although you don't talk, there are movements that mean certain things, bits of business, ways of conveying emotions and putting over a feeling. When you're walking from Center Stage to Stage Left, you should be aware of how you feel it mentally and how you're going to do that turn before it's ever done, so that it is done well. You're always ahead of yourself, so you'll complete every move with a feeling of continuity. If a model will try a turn without thinking much about it beforehand, it will show in the way she does it, and fare poorly, compared with an emotionally and mentally completed plan. You should always be ahead of yourself, as if you were following a shadow. This will have an effect on your modeling.

Let's take examples of some costumes and see if you can create a feeling that shows. Your walk must be paced correctly, and the use of your hands must be elegant, as we discussed in a previous chapter.

YOU ARE MODELING	YOU SHOULD FEEL
A flowing peignoir set	Tenderness, softness, femininity, love.
A man-tailored Spanish style	Gusto, spirit, alertness, ease.
Wild hostess pajamas	Inspiration, a tremendous amount of confidence, humor, self-assurance, a great love of life, and a definite cordiality.

British tailored suit	Deep sense of satisfaction, inspiration for outdoors, a bit more briskness, a zest.
A long, beaded evening gown	Complete control, feeling of being loved and admired, self-confidence, knowledge that it's right for you.
A flowing chiffon	An airy lightness, warmth, knowing you're all woman.
A multicolored crazy-quilt patterned evening culotte	Zest and confidence, a breezy feeling that you can "get away with it."

Try very hard to capture the mood of the costume you're wearing. It should show and be expressed in the way you model it. Above all, your attitude that the costume is just right for you is important. If you feel right in it and make yourself think so, you will show that feeling. Someone watching you will feel the same way, that she will be right in it too, and this sells the garment.

Your walk should have an alertness about it, but the turns should be smooth and fairly slow compared with your walk. You are turning to *show* a garment, and if you whirl around you won't show it well. Your audience will only think of it as an attractive turn rather than viewing something you're trying to sell. Always remember, you are trying to sell clothes. Show them beautifully.

There may be professional models reading this book who will possibly see something new and unfamiliar, and wonder, "Now, why does she think she's able to do all this?"

I've traveled widely in the fashion world and viewed fashion shows in San Francisco, Los Angeles, New York, in all the chic fashion centers, and seen all the top models. I've seen and worked with the cream of the European models, from France, Japan, Italy, England, Switzerland. I've taken and used their techniques. I've chosen the most beautiful things they do and incorporated them into a compact way of doing them.

You will find your New York models working with the methods I'm telling you about now. These are the top models, and they, in turn, have learned from the European girls. I have avoided some of the European things that are being done because, possibly, they are a little too extreme. One girl conceivably might be able to carry it off, but it wouldn't be standard enough to benefit the majority. The ideas we are giving are good basic modeling techniques that are beautiful to view and excellent training. You will look right doing them.

A model who is seriously interested in improving herself will go to fashion shows. She will watch professionals, and maybe pick up one small bit of information that is suitable for her. It may be a hand position, a turn of the head, anything that is beautiful. What is going to be beautiful? What will sell clothes? What will look right on a stage?

If you learn all of this, you will be able to work anywhere in the world. You must be able to adjust. Whenever a designer tells you to walk differently, take larger steps, drop your shoulders a bit more, don't smile, do smile, whatever it is, you should be able to adjust to it. Even though you know it's usually done another way, if a designer wants something done especially his way — possibly to try to prove a mood or feeling for his clothes — you don't question it or say anything about it. You do what he tells you. Be adaptable, be pleasant, and do what he wants you to do.

You must be able to talk to people. Let your eyes sparkle. Look people directly in the eyes. Be extremely self-confident. Notice the clear, direct, confident appearance a photographic model can give to a camera. This is what you must give to your audience.

First of all, a magnetic personality shows enthusiasm. You can't sparkle for someone else if you're not sparkling for yourself. You should have a zest for the little things in life as well as the big things. The enthusiasm we have in our everyday life will come through. It is very rare to find a model who is dull and blasé in real life and who can come onstage and suddenly be magnetic. This really has to be a part of you.

You sparkle. You have tremendous enthusiasm for whatever you put on. You create a love and a feeling for whatever you are doing. Whatever your assignment may be, this inner glow must come through.

This inner sparkle is developed with your inner character. It may be just a great big bore to someone else, but this is the greatest youth-giving device a woman can give herself. It's admittedly very difficult to do at certain times in your life, but you must create an optimistic outlook. You must have a good philosophy of life to truly have a magnetic, irresistible personality that people are drawn to.

You're not interested in yourself, necessarily, but in what's going on around you, in what you're doing. It's an appreciation of just every minute of your life. It's the joy you feel at the sight of a sliver of new moon in a dark blue sky, the pleasure you get from the liquid notes of a single bird singing in the morning, the way you feel when a fresh breeze ruffles your hair. It may be something as prosaic as your delight when a library finally has the book you've wanted for weeks! You have to be aware of and alive to everything around you, and this means people and things.

You can develop this inner incandescence, but you can work on the outer you in a more tangible way. We can look at ourselves and know that we can develop and do exercises, to help ourselves. But you must have your inner exercise daily too, and that is to love life and wake up feeling wonderful. This means that you must do everything in moderation.

You're surely not going to show a magnetic personality if you stayed up all night! You are going to feel and show that you're tired. It will be obvious in your voice as well as in your face. Remember that a model on a runway or a stage has to pantomime, in a sense. You are not talking up there, but you literally have to tell people you love what you're doing. Your expression must show it. Your body movements must be just right, but it's the facial expression that is so important.

EXERCISES FOR FACIAL EXPRESSION

To create good muscle control in the face, you have to learn to smile and hold an expression. I know, you always thought smiling comes naturally. It does, and it doesn't. In modeling, you have to work at it. Now, let's begin.

1. Stand in front of a mirror. Close your eyes. Relax your face and tongue. Let your whole body relax completely. Open your eyes. Look into them very carefully. Look at your face. Everything is relaxed. You look rather dull, in fact. Now, don't grin. I know you're tempted, but this is a serious matter of comparing. I wonder if you're aware of how many people sit around and look as if they're entirely bored with life with this completely relaxed look? You can't look like this and come through radiant.

So, let's switch it now. Close your eyes. Relax your mouth, and your facial muscles, and your tongue. Your lip area must be very soft and relaxed. Now pretend that someone has just put a beautiful rose under your nose and you're smelling it. Smell it now. Mm-m-m-m! It's a beautiful rose. Do you notice, when you smell the rose, the lift of the muscles at the outer corners of the mouth?

Open your eyes. You smell that rose. Hold that expression. Do you see the difference in your eyes? You should see it in your facial expression, too. This is the beginning, so you can see that it is an inner feeling. It can't just come from merely lifting the corners of the mouth. It must come from within.

Now, as you talk with people, learn to lean forward with this rather interested expression. The corners of your mouth will be lifted, and there will be an excitement in your eyes, as if you were clinging to every word your partner is saying. You just can't wait to hear more!

Try it. Experiment with it. You'll develop much more charm because people will feel flattered that you're interested in them. Basically, of course, I feel that you should really have a desire to look at people and listen to them and know they have something to offer. Be excited about what goes on in the world, so that it shows in your face and your eyes.

2. This is the hardest exercise, because it is true muscle training. Step in front of a mirror now, but after a while you won't have to use it. It might be a good idea for you to be alone when you're doing this. We do it in class and it makes everybody laugh, but you really should practice this alone because you must be completely uninhibited and realize that you will develop a smile by exercising.

Open your mouth as wide as you can, to stretch the muscles on either side. Open it wide; stretch it. Now pull your mouth way over to the left and stretch the side of your face as far over as you can. Hold it for a count of 6. Now over to the other side, and stretch it. It's an isometric type of exercise. Stretch it and hold it. Open your mouth again, and stretch it. Now pucker it, as if you were trying to touch your nose with your lips.

You now have exercised your lips by opening, puckering, pulling to the side. If you do not smile easily or readily, and the muscles have not been used, it's difficult to smile. You must relax the muscles and work them so that it's easier to smile. Do this again. Now notice how much easier it is to smile because you've worked the muscles. You've actually *stretched* them.

All right. Now we're going to learn how to *hold* a smile. First for one minute, and then I want it worked up to three minutes. By learning to smile, we work the muscles and strengthen them. Before each exercise, you should stretch the muscles around your face.

3. Looking into your mirror, stretch your mouth into as full a grin as you can. It should be a really tight grin, to show and expose all your teeth. Your lower lip should be touching just the edge of your upper teeth. All your teeth show. Press your tongue to the back of your upper teeth, ever so gently. This will control the smile up to a point. Hold this for one minute. Really hold it firmly. Don't let it relax. You'll find that your face may be sore.

This should be done for one minute a day until it becomes very easy, then you may increase it by thirty seconds. You should be able to hold a smile for three minutes, if you're really working in earnest. Then the muscles start lifting. It's a marvelous facial toner. You'll look younger for a much longer time if you learn to smile and to lift the muscles of your face.

HEAD MOVEMENTS

Here are some points to be careful about regarding head movements. Don't jerk your head or be too quick with it. Your head should move with ease. Your eyes and your mouth and your facial expression change, and your head moves smoothly. You learn to blink your eyes. A girl who stares gives a static expression. I have seen this onstage. A model won't blink her eyes and does her routine glassy-eyed. It leaves something to be desired.

If you blink your eyes, you'll find that there's a little bit of warmth and response. It's an "I-like-you" kind of thing. In class, I have my students walk toward a mirror, stare straight into it, looking at their reflected faces as another person would see them. Then they'll blink their eyes and mentally say, "I like you." They can see the effect themselves. This is what you want to convey to your customers—"I like you."

I'm forever trying to have the model realize that she is in a position where she's very often envied, with everyone just looking for a chance to criticize. To become an exceptional model, you should be warm and alive and do your job well, *and look as if you like your audience.* You'll have to practice this with your co-workers, as well as with the people to whom you're projecting.

Teach your head to be quiet. Your eyes and your mouth are what show the enthusiasm and the magnetic part of you. Let them create an expression that's alive. Sparkle. Make your eyes open a little wider sometimes, and then blink.

EYE EXERCISES

You should give your eyes some exercise, too. I believe it's a good idea to exercise your eyes when you turn the lights out at night. You're in the dark, and that's a good time to do eye exercises. Open them as wide as you can, and roll them in a slow circle, or down to the side and then up. Open them wide and stretch them. Now reverse it. Go seven times in one direction and seven times the other way.

Then squeeze your eyes shut. This utilizes the same principle involved when you squeeze your hand to bring the blood up for a blood count. You squeeze your eyes and you help them. It brings the blood up to your eyes. It feeds them, in a manner of speaking.

Squeeze them, open them, stretch them, roll them. Over and over. Do this in the dark. In the daytime, look as far into the distance as you can, then look at something close by, then far into the distance again. Any exercises that an optometrist would give you would be excellent, but these are good ones which you can do every day.

Remember, blink your eyes, show interest, lean forward. The truly magnetic person isn't interested in telling you her troubles. She is interested in listening to *you* in a sympathetic manner or with enthusiasm, and she can be truly happy for another person's good fortune. Develop this quality.

I always notice that the students who have taken dramatic lessons come through so much better because in acting classes you must use your muscles and your expression areas. Drama students are able to adopt a mood because they are trained. I urgently suggest that you join a small acting class. Don't be afraid to use expression. Let it come through. Many models have gone into the acting field; modeling has been a stepping stone into the acting world. As successful models, they have more doors open to them. With acting, there is so much competition that if you already have all the attributes of a model and keep up with your drama training, you'll have something extra going for you.

INNER BEAUTY

Your personality should reflect your inner beauty. We're always hearing about the golden rule, and probably you're tired of hearing about it. It's much easier to say "Follow the golden rule" than to actually do it. Yet, there are so many areas in your personality to which the golden rule applies. You must have a sense of humor, be able to admit mistakes, and not be supersensitive. You might even be big enough to admit mistakes you're not sure you've made, if they're not too important.

KEEP YOUR GROOMING PERFECT

You must have good grooming habits. Know that you look well and take time for yourself so that your personality shines through. How can you have a beautiful personality if you know you've neglected any area of yourself? Subconsciously, you won't come through. In every way—whether in dress or manners or eating habits—a model must try to make every area her best. Admit you're not perfect, but always keep trying to be.

Ask for criticism. Thank anyone for it. If you're inwardly not quite sure about accepting it, go to someone else. Go to someone you admire

and whose opinion you value. Weigh this carefully. It doesn't mean
that everybody's criticism will be valid, but weigh it for yourself in
an intelligent manner.

ACCEPTING AND GIVING CRITICISM

You'll find when you work with a model agency or other models
that you'll have to learn to accept criticism and ideas. I have found
that many models resent this. I may say that the color of her hair isn't
quite right, or her eye makeup. This may be just my opinion but I, as
a director, must keep up on things, and if my model isn't selling one
way, I have to try another way. Maybe the color of her hair isn't right,
or her attitude or her expression. It could be any of these things and a
host of others. Is she dressed right?

A model should always look like a model. We often hear that photographic models are more casual, or that they have a more natural,
somewhat unkempt look. This is the way they want many photographic
models, but a fashion model must look like a fashion model at all times.
It must become second nature to you. It's just as easy to put all of yourself together the correct way and walk out of the house so that people
who see you know you always look right, and they will enjoy the things
you do.

When I speak of criticism—asking for it, accepting it, and thanking someone for it whether you like it or not—I mean you must be truly
sincere about it. Now let's look at the other side of it. Are you criticizing others?

Models do occasionally help one another, but sometimes this is
resented. If you're truly trying to be helpful, be careful how you voice
your criticism. Rather than say you don't care for a girl's hairstyle,
say, "Oh, look at this hairstyle. I think it would be great for you. You
could wear it beautifully. You can wear many hairstyles well, but I'd
love to see you in this. Why don't you give it a try?"

You see, you're not literally criticizing her hairstyle. You're
merely suggesting that she try this one. This gives her the impression that you're helping her.

For example, notice the new hairstyles. There is almost no teasing at all. Basically, teasing is out. Still, you may find a girl stubbornly
staying with the teased-out styles. In the past—and this will happen,
no matter in which era we live—there have been women who take
three years to accept a new idea, and then cling to that one for another
three years, long after the fashion has faded away.

It will always be this way, but when you see a new idea or someone suggests it, don't cling to the old ideas and think you can't change

or look different. Remember, I am speaking now to models or people who want to look like models. You have to learn to accept the fact that you're expected to look different, to have the latest look in beauty as well as fashion. You may look strange to the eyes of others, even to yourself, but it's a new designer's idea, and you're his showcase.

It would be a stagnant world indeed in the fashion field if we didn't have things to draw our attention because they are new. It's an ever-changing look. Surprisingly enough, some girls can change a look and still keep their individual style. For instance, if you think you're a sleek girl, think how many different ways you can create a sleek look. You can style your hair in evening do's, daytime coifs, short cuts, long cuts. You can go through many different looks, but your hair need never have a really curly look.

Getting back to criticism, be careful how you voice it. You want to be liked. Don't be a faultfinder. Be helpful, be tactful, and be intuitive to the needs of others. Hopefully, as a woman, you will have this feeling within yourself. Calling a spade a spade is an old cliché, and is often an excuse for plain rudeness, but everyone doesn't feel this way. Be kind, as if you might hurt people's feelings and are determined to be tactful. You'll be far better off. Without being hypocritical, sometimes you're better off just being quiet, smiling, and being complimentary. You'll certainly be safer!

In your business, where you must defer to so many people who may be over you, you have to accept criticism. You accept it from the photographer, the coordinator, the director, or the agency. It's the greatest thing in the world if you can realize that they're all trying to do things for your benefit. They are not against you. They are *for* you.

PUTTING YOURSELF OVER

Let's go back and add up some of the things which make a model's personality come through. Your facial expression, which involves your eyes, your mouth, the muscles of your face, and an inner glow, which is personal adjustment and a philosophy of life that is healthy. Personality goes deeper and farther and includes the inner portion of your manner, your conversation, and your voice. You may never have to talk onstage, yet in meeting people who may hire you, your voice may tip the balance in your favor. If you're going to do any talking in salon or tearoom modeling, your voice is most important. All of these facets are part of your personality, and you'll have to practice before you acquire them.

Make it a point, as of now, that with every person you meet, you will be the first to smile and say hello. Whether it's on the street or on the telephone, smile and say, "Hello," and make that "o" go up, so that it's a delightful sound. Not just a limp "hel-lo." Smile, and the "o" goes up. Feel the difference?

Do not complain. Accept. Listen carefully. Listen to the problems of others and don't relate yours unless you do so in a humorous manner. Use your own good judgment.

Your personality also involves the visible you. This means your hair, your figure, your wardrobe, the way you're coordinated, your tangible poise. What do people see visually? If all of these are functioning as a coordinated whole, you will be far ahead of the game.

Know what's going on in the world. Read the front pages. You don't have to be an expert on political science or heart transplants, but you should be able to recognize names and places that are in the news. The more interests you have in life, the better the personality you will create for yourself. For some people, this is very difficult to do but you must try to develop it. The more knowledge you have, the more personality you'll have, and you'll be more charming because you can talk to more people on their level.

You can be most attractive and be a model, but because of this people are often frightened of you. They're afraid to approach you, but if you show an interest in them and make them talk about themselves, this helps you. You become more charming and beautiful.

At times you may have to pretend a poised and confident look, but the more you pretend and know you have done well for yourself, the more it will be true. You will cement the inner feeling that you do have this confidence, and look it. This is what we want, so don't be afraid to recognize that you are pretending sometimes, but that it will come true.

Work on this and on every other idea you've learned that will bring out your personal magnetism and, believe me, it all will come true. You'll be poised and beautiful, and you'll absolutely radiate charm!

12

HOW TO PRODUCE YOUR OWN FASHION SHOW

PLANNING IS HALF THE BATTLE

A successful fashion show doesn't just happen. It must be well planned from start to finish. When a group of women get together to plan a money-making event, which is what they usually have in mind with a fashion show, they frequently haven't the slightest idea where or how to begin. They have two alternatives. They can either blunder through (with the best will in the world), or hire professional help.

Sometimes, out of sheer luck and with the help of some heretofore unsuspected genius, a beautiful production will result from the first method. More often, it will be obviously amateur. Hiring professional help will result in a professional production, but the money so invested will have to be siphoned off from whatever has been earned for the organization. Hobson's choice? Not really. There is one other alternative. The women can work with a plan which has been geared specifically to their particular needs. This section has been prepared to assist groups and organizations with the business of putting on a perfect fashion show.

This can be done by an organization (charitable or social), a dress shop, a church, a school, or another group. Your planning will actually cover two categories: administration and fashion show production.

Administration involves the backstage workings of the entire endeavor. Under this heading come most, sometimes all, of your committees. It covers tickets, publicity, prizes, hostesses, wardrobe women, and so on.

219

Fashion Show Production, as its name implies, will cover selection of a theme, preparing the program, choosing the models, the clothes, and the accessories. In short, all the drama of a fashion show from rehearsals to the finale.

Since you should have all your administration details ironed out before you attempt anything else, let's have first things first.

PLANNING YOUR ADMINISTRATION

Within an organization, many will have to give up much of their time and/or talent. Before any of you touch a pencil or lift a telephone, you must select your time, pick your place, and choose your committees.

Time

The first thing to be considered is the time you plan to have your showing. Always plan for an early spring or fall showing. You never plan a fashion show when all the sales are going on. Merchants want to show new merchandise early to stimulate buying for the coming season. The committee in charge of selecting the fashions should check with the stores whose clothes they plan to use, and make sure when their merchandise will be available.

Before you do even this, it's a wise idea to call your local Chamber of Commerce and find out what fashion shows and other city events are planned during the same month. It is always good judgment to have your show on a day that is clear of other events. You will lose out on revenue if you find yourself competing with a function that your potential patrons will find equally — or more — attractive than yours.

August, September, and October are best for a fall showing. November and December are a little late, but a showing can be planned for then. There are fashion shows in December, but people are buying for Christmas, we hope, before December.

March, April, and May are for your spring and summer fashion shows. In some areas, February could be used, but stores might not have all their spring merchandise in. They may, but you'll have to check this out with the stores. June and July are rather late, as they are sale months. January and February are sale months also.

Once you have established your date, planning two months ahead, I would say, is ideal and should give you enough time. Just to keep you on the calendar for your own city, though, it doesn't hurt to plan six months in advance. *This is most important.*

Place

Most fashion shows are held in dining rooms of hotels, and a luncheon is part of the package. You can also hold a fashion show in a clubroom or a special room in a hotel, a cocktail room or small ballroom, or a restaurant. Perhaps one of the theatre owners in your city will let you use his facilities. You could use the community theatre, or if it's a school presentation, you have the school auditorium.

Once you've decided on the place, it's up to the proper committee to make sure that the location is available for the chosen date, that facilities will be ample for your needs, what *exactly* is provided by the management, and that the contracts, or letters of agreement, are gone over carefully before signing.

Committees

Next, you select your committees, and each committee should have a cochairman and someone to assist her. When all committees are chosen, the Ways and Means chairman has jurisdiction over all committees and keeps in touch with all of them. All reports are given to her, and she should keep a chart of the calls that come in and what is being done.

There should be regular periodic meetings of individual committees, as well as meetings of committee chairmen. Each chairman and cochairman should know her own responsibilities.

You will need a committee for each of these:

1. Publicity
2. Program
3. Table decorations
4. Tickets
5. Backstage (lights, props, decorations, etc.)
6. Prizes

Besides these committees, you will need:

1. Fashion coordinator
2. Commentator (sometimes the same person as the coordinator)
3. Stage manager and stagehands
4. Musician or musicians
5. Spotlight man and electricians
6. Sound man (microphone)
7. Wardrobe women
8. Hostesses

TICKET COMMITTEE

When your theme has been established, as well as the time, the date, and the beneficiary of the charity, it's time to think of tickets. Your publicity, of course, and other facets of the show planning are all going on simultaneously by now. Your ticket committee chairman will see that the tickets are printed.

You should have an approximate goal of the number of tickets you're going to sell. Say, for instance, that a group has one hundred women and it sets a goal for each to sell four tickets. You will plan for four hundred. A smaller group may have only twenty-five women, and they will sell ten tickets each. They'll have two hundred fifty. Whatever it may be, each organization sets a goal for what it is going to establish in the ticket sales.

You also will have to have tickets made up for your raffle, unless you use the admission tickets for this. Guests should write their names on the stubs. You'll make extra revenue by selling raffle tickets at your fashion show. These tickets could be cheaper bought in quantity, three for 25¢, or an extra ticket if a dollar's worth is purchased. (Be sure to include "Donation" on the ticket when specifying the price. Check this, to make sure that your organization will not have to pay tax on your receipts.)

How to Determine the Price of a Ticket

The price to establish for a fashion-show admission will be determined by the cost of the luncheon. The committee member who reports on this will obtain several prices, and they will vary. A more elaborate luncheon will cost more, and the time of the year makes a difference, too. This is where it becomes personalized. For example, though, we'll take $3.50 as the price for a light luncheon. You can add a dollar over that. Then you can get an idea of what you will take in. You can add $2, if you like. It's up to you. Just do what you want to, and what you think the traffic will bear. Can you sell enough tickets at such a price? It's a personal thing.

If there are no expenses involved, anything you get over and above the cost of the luncheon will be clear profit for your cause. Usually, however, there is a certain amount of expenses involved. You can't get *everything* donated. Tickets, for instance, may end up costing you upward of $50. You might bring down the price of the tickets—or maybe even get them for nothing—if you put the printer's name on the back of the tickets. There are generally at least two hundred women attending, and he will get free publicity. Of course the chances that many or any of the women in your audience will ever need a commercial printer are fairly remote, but just don't remind him! Or you can ask a business firm which wants the publicity to advertise on the back of the tickets and pay for the printing.

All other committees should take note of this. There are ways of getting people to donate products or services by promising the donors free publicity — in the program and possibly through other means.

If the printers don't consider this worth their while, you might try to have the dress shop (whose clothes you're showing) donate money for the tickets. If they won't go for it, try a furniture store, or any store in the city or in the neighborhood. Just tell them, "You buy the tickets and we'll see that you get publicity on each ticket and on the program as well." Use your imagination on getting as much as possible for a charity show free.

Getting back to your luncheon prices, if the luncheon is $3.50 you might add $1.50 and get a final price of $5 per ticket. In some communities, this is considered nominal, and in others some people might think it's a great deal of money. You'll have to judge carefully here, and take into account the type of women who will be attending, and how much you think they can afford. Your object is to make money for your organization, but if you price your tickets out of reach you'll find yourself playing to an empty house. Think this over and discuss it with your committee first (perhaps with the entire group) before you decide on your final figure.

When you have arrived at that figure and know how much more you will be charging above the luncheon price and how many tickets you expect to sell, then you will know how much money you can expect to earn. If you charge a dollar over, and four hundred women attend, you will have earned $400, if you have no other expenses. If you have other expenses, you will have to deduct them from that $400 total. It's up to you to keep the expenses down.

PUBLICITY COMMITTEE

Your publicity chairman should have an assistant. Either or both of them should be qualified to write releases and prepare a good publicity program. Possibly one could be an expert at writing releases and the other proficient as an "idea" person. A good publicity job will include sending out press releases, contacting local radio and TV personalities, having posters made up and seeing that they are placed strategically around town, and having invitations sent to people you think would be interested.

Preparing a Press Release

An effective press release should convey the pertinent facts about the fashion show in as short and interesting a manner as possible. Always type your news carefully and double-space. Keep your release short, never longer than two pages, but one and a half are usually ample. Reporters, columnists, and editors are busy people and they don't want to have to wade through pages and pages of prose to get to the heart of the matter. Another thing that editors dislike is receiving releases on long, legal-size sheets of paper. Most newspaper and magazine filing cabinet drawers are still 9 by 12 and, rather than go through the bother of folding or crumpling, the editor, or his secretary, may send your precious release to that universal filing cabinet, the waste basket. This isn't usual, but it has been known to happen!

If you think your *important* news is longer than two pages, there's no reason why you can't send several releases, reasonably spaced apart. Or send two releases in the same envelope; one will be a regular release explaining things and the other will be a fact sheet. Your fact sheet can list—in one-two-three form—some of the important points of your show. You could list some of the models' names this way, or facts about, say, a special new fabric you're using in the show, or brief bios (biographies) of different members of the organization. Needless to say, these must be interesting people, either socially prominent, or unusual scholastically, or professionally important.

Be sure your names and places are *correctly spelled*. You know the old saying, "I don't care what you say about me, but make sure you spell my name right." I wouldn't go quite that far, but you know what I mean. People can be most unreasonable about having their names misspelled, so do it right. If you're not sure, phone and have it spelled, then double-check.

Remember the five w's in your publicity—who, where, when, why, and what. It works for newspapermen and it will work for you. If you cover all five thoroughly and to the point, you'll have a good press release.

Get your news in a week early. If necessary, get it in two weeks ahead. Your society or women's page editor plans her work in advance, and you may miss out by being possibly three or four hours too late. If you live in a small city, the society editor on your local newspaper will be glad to help you, but her time is precious so don't take up too much of it. Have your material prepared. Let her know the date you plan for your fashion show and ask her by what date she wants your publicity submitted.

You should plan to have something in the paper every week—sometimes twice a week—for at least a month before the show. Just little things, but keep interest alive and people aware of you. You might send a picture of the shop owner and a model, or one of the models alone, or some of the committeewomen. You might remember, too, that a city editor always has an eye for a pretty girl and a clever caption! Find out how many photographs your editor can use.

Sometimes in certain locales, some newspapers will give you a whole society page, maybe even send out their own photographer, especially if it's a charity show for which the women are donating their time.

At the fashion show, there should always be a table set aside for the press. Write an invitation and send it to the society editors of every newspaper to which you've submitted releases, as well as to radio and TV people. These people should be your guests at the press table, and a formal invitation must be mailed to them.

Radio and TV Publicity

Call your local radio station or stations, and tell them that you plan a fashion show. Ask them to announce the date and the charity it will benefit. They will usually cooperate if you plan an interesting presentation. Large network stations, of course, may not be able to help as far as announcing your show. Often their programming just doesn't work this way. They may, however, have one or two informal talk shows where such an announcement could be made. Find out if this is possible. Another possibility with a large network, if you have a personality or a gimmick that is sufficiently intriguing, is to contact the News Department and they may send a reporter out.

Your local TV station should be visited. Try to get on their interview shows. Have an interesting presentation ready. Women are always fascinated with clothes. Excite them about the fashions you'll be presenting, without actually giving the show away, and feature a shop whose clothes people are interested in seeing. Play up the new season ahead. Everybody's eager to know what's coming up for the next season, especially something they haven't seen yet. Make it sound gay and stimulating and worthwhile coming to see. Women love to see new fashions.

You'll have a better chance at network publicity, as well as having an added attraction for your guests, if you can wangle an outstanding personality to visit your showing, possibly even act as master of ceremonies. He might just do it for sweet charity. If you can't get a star of the first magnitude, perhaps you can get a minor celebrity — singer or nightclub entertainer — in your town who would be glad to help you. He may come in just for an hour or less, donating his time to the cause, and introduce the commentator and open the show. You must let the public know you're going to have an outstanding fashion show, and that they'll miss the event of the year if they don't come.

Posters

You should have posters in various store windows around your town, wherever they would do the most good and, naturally, in the windows of the dress shop that will be presenting the fashions.

You can get the posters made in art classes. Ask your local art students to use this idea as a project. High schools and university art departments will often cooperate, but you must let them know far enough in advance. The posters should look professional. It is important to keep costs down as much as possible, especially if it is for charity, but your art students should be able to make a good job of the posters.

You may have a talented girl within your own organization who can do this. But the point is—get it done. Then get your posters out and around, at least two to three weeks early. And don't forget the window—or showcase—of the place where your fashion show will be held.

Formal Invitations

There is one more form of publicity that might be very effective for your purposes. This is the formal invitation. Sometimes your group might have a list of people who would be reasonably certain to want to attend. You can send formal invitations, simply worded, giving the date, time, price, and the charity to benefit.

Example:
You are cordially invited to attend
(name of group)   on (date)
Presentation of Spring Fashions to be
held at _____ o'clock in the
dining room of (name of place)
Luncheon $2.50   R.S.V.P. (phone number)
Name of Charity

These personal invitations can do very well with groups. Just be sure that you don't get them mixed up with the invitations you send to the press and to anyone you want to honor with a free ticket. These would be entirely different invitations, *with no mention of price.*

TABLE DECORATIONS AND STAGE SETTING

Usually you work around the theme of your show, as far as decorations are concerned. The chairman who, with her committee, decorates the stage might very well be the one who does the tables. After all, how many women do you have who can donate the time?

Your local artist may come up with some clever ideas. Your local florist, for publicity, may do something for you. Most of the time, however, the women end up doing the whole job themselves. Many interesting and artistic things can be done with plastic cutouts and art paper, but keep in mind that it will all take extra time, so plan on it.

If it's a spring event, you might use a small nosegay for a centerpiece on each table, or a floral piece denoting the theme.

Table Decorations

If favors are planned, or some gifts which are usually giveaways by the local drugstore or cosmetic counter of a shop as a goodwill gesture, they should be prepackaged and placed at each place setting on the tables when they are decorated.

Find out from the maître d' what time is most convenient for decorating the tables. As the waiters are setting the tables for the luncheon, your committee can do the decorating.

Setting the Stage

There are various things that can be done here. Your stage chairman can call furniture companies and offer them publicity on the program if they will deliver certain props that would contribute to a nice setting. In the summertime, it can be lawn furniture, sometimes fountains.

Telephone calls to check on work progress are necessary. Use your telephone for every phase of your planning. It will save you many trips.

Call a landscape architect and offer him publicity if he'll send shrubs or bushes and trees, and place them in certain spots. Check these out and make sure they're delivered early, and that the people know where to deliver them.

Dress Delivery

While I'm on that subject, I might add that it's very important to let the dress shop know *exactly* where they're to deliver the clothes.

A sheet or some sort of covering should be provided for the floor, so that girls stepping into and out of garments will not soil the clothing. A mirror or two, a chair for every girl, and a table should be provided. These are all marvelous, if you can get them. A full-length mirror is ideal. If you can manage this, have a long table, with a chair and a space, about 24 inches, for each girl all down the line. This would be perfect, but many a fashion show has been held where a girl had only a chair to work from.

You'll need clothes racks and extra hangers where girls can hang their own clothes. There should be one woman in charge of this, with a number of wardrobe women (as we call them) helping her.

HOSTESSES AND PRIZE COMMITTEE

You must have hostesses at the luncheon to see that each guest signs her ticket. You must have pen and pencil ready, and have the hostesses greet the guests and help seat them.

As far as a seating plan is concerned, I usually find it's best to go by the old "first come-first served" method, but the one table you will have to reserve will be for the press, and these invitations are handled by the Publicity Committee, as suggested above.

You will probably find it best, except for the women who are literally working for the show, that no other person should receive a free ticket. Only press people, and that should be standard procedure. Otherwise you'll be giving too many things away. Just because a member works hard on a show doesn't mean she's entitled to a free ticket for a friend. She'll have to buy it.

In some cases, a member must buy her own ticket, to support the charity. I don't think it's a bad idea. If you're going to support a charity, support it all the way. Your work is just an extra contribution. You're going to see the show and eat the luncheon, so you will pay for it as for any other entertainment. It's up to each individual organization to decide the policy.

Your hostesses will also help with the prizes. They will sell the raffle tickets, if this is done during the luncheon, and later will help get the prizes to the winners.

Offering prizes at a fashion show, or any other function, always adds an extra fillip to the proceedings and attracts more patrons. You will need a prize committee to collect the items to be given away. Your hostesses will attend to the mechanics of the actual raffle. Possibly your hostesses might be members of the prize committee. You'll have to work this out for yourselves.

You very probably will be selling raffle tickets while guests are being seated, but some groups prefer not to. Again, it's a matter of individual choice.

For the giving away of prizes, some people like to break the fashion show in the middle—offering the girls a little rest—and have the raffle in the interval between. I personally don't like this. A better break, if you want to have one, would be to insert a bit of entertainment. There might be someone who's going to sing for you, someone to tell a joke or two, or a personality you might want to introduce. A little lightness between the fashions is fine. It's still entertainment.

Using the break for raffling the prizes is different. Somehow, after all the prizes have been announced and the fashion showing comes back, you have lost a certain flavor by stopping for something as far removed from the mood as a raffle. Except for a break for entertainment, if desired, I think it's nice to be able to go on with the showing. It can be done, though, so it's up to the women to decide. It has been done both ways.

Wherever you decide to hold your raffle—in the middle of your show or at the end—the cardinal rule is: *don't let it drag.* Have your box for tickets ready. A pretty little hatbox will do, or any receptacle you can whirl, and someone can reach in and pick out a ticket. Know in advance who's going to come up and assist with this. Have her close to the steps so that she can step right up and assist you.

Call the numbers off, and your hostesses can deliver the packages to the winners, rather than have each winner get out of her seat to walk all the way down the length of the room and then up onto the stage. Another way is to get her name, call it, have her stand, and take the prize to her. During the time one hostess is taking a prize to its winner, another number can be called and another hostess can be on her way. This will make the raffle proceedings much more efficient than some I have seen.

It's a long drag to wait for a woman to walk up, give her name, wait for a handclap, and then walk back to her seat. Then you call another name. Fifteen minutes can go by in this procedure. Whether you know it or not, a woman really doesn't like to sit for more than an hour when she's all dressed up, wearing a tight girdle.

A good fashion show should not last longer than an hour at the most. The audience has already been sitting for a half-hour eating, and at times it's closer to forty-five minutes or an hour. Let's say the appointed hour is 12 noon. Luncheon is served at 12:30; it takes that long for guests to be seated. The fashion show starts at 1. By the time 2 o'clock rolls around, guests are ready to get up and move around a bit. So, plan your timing.

As people are winning prizes, it's pleasant to have a little musical background. I feel that if a woman is going to have to go up to get her prize, she feels awkward walking the full length of the room in silence. Be sure that the musicians play a peppy tune—a "Here-Comes-the-Winner" sort of thing.

Don't always wrap the prizes. The audience likes to see what they are.

Keep a list of the winners' names. Have each hostess who delivers a prize write the name down and send it up to the chairman, who then will be able to announce the winners.

PROGRAM COMMITTEE

Your fashion coordinator, the M.C. (whoever he is), and the head chairman should get together and make up an exact program, closely following the printed program, which is given to your guests.

These programs can be printed or they may be mimeographed. I've seen some fine mimeographed programs, with art work included. It will probably make more work and won't be as professional as a printer's program, but if you're watching the budget it can be very satisfactory. I have had high-school students do a lovely fashion show, with the students making up the programs and mimeographing them on school machines.

Always double-check your programs to make sure that all the names are spelled correctly and that you have not forgotten anyone who should be mentioned. Be extra careful of this when making up your programs. It's very disconcerting to a person to donate something or do something free in a fashion show for publicity, and then not have credit for it in the program! This is one of the most horrible crimes in the public-relations world. At best, you'll have some hurt feelings, and at worst, you'll never get anything from that particular source again.

A double caution—see that everyone's name is spelled right and listed in its proper place. Check your copy several times, and with several people. Read it *before* it goes to the printer (or mimeograph machine); *after* it comes back in proof form; and the *final copy* when it's ready for reproduction. Check and double-check and, remember, give credit where credit is due!

WARDROBE COMMITTEE

Wardrobe women are an important part of any fashion show, doubly so when the models are amateurs and do not dress as quickly as professionals. You should have a chairman backstage, with as many women to help as necessary in assisting the girls with their changes. This will vary. If all the girls are amateurs, it would be wise to have *one* person assisting every *two* models, providing you have enough space and enough volunteers.

Another duty that falls to the wardrobe committee is to see that all garments are pressed. The shop should send them to you already pressed. This is their responsibility. Remind them that you want to show their clothes to the best advantage.

Models must be reminded—and this is most important—that they are *never* to sit in any of the clothes they wear for the show. They also must be very careful that the clothes are put back on the hangers. If there's no time for the model to do this herself, she can hand them to a wardrobe woman.

Your backstage wardrobe women should always be certain that clothes are unzipped or unsnapped. Be sure that tags are pinned *under* a garment. It's part of their job to notice these things. They should know who their models are and be ready to assist them. As soon as a model comes in, the wardrobe woman will unzip her and help her to step out of the clothes. She should be ready with the next dress the model is to wear.

The wardrobe woman should know the lineup of the clothes as well as the model. She checks the model very carefully, always working with her. It shouldn't take a model longer than a minute to get dressed. You can allow more time, but a good model can get dressed backstage in a minute, even faster, if everything is ready. We've timed it. Two to three minutes are ample.

The Music

Music for your production is most important. You cannot present a good show without it.

If you have to use someone in your group who is talented and will donate a little time, do try to find someone who has enough instinctive feeling to switch the tempo of the music as the mood of the costume changes. If you have a professional pianist, or an organist, or an accordionist, or any musician, be sure that he knows he has to switch tempos. If you have a bigger budget, you can consider hiring a three-piece group; even a larger one, if the showing is very elaborate.

Whatever your final choice, the musician, or leader of the musical group, must be supplied with a lineup sheet, which we'll talk about later. He must know beforehand that he has to look at it, so it will give him a general idea. He must know the theme of the show in advance so that he can select the appropriate music.

You should know what your opening and closing songs will be. Usually it's a gay, lively tune for your opening, and something that will send them out humming for your closing. The music must tie in with the clothes being shown.

You can, if you're imaginative, work fashion-show music around what a girl is wearing. If you're not inventive enough, it would depend on the musician. Really work on planning your musical accompaniment, and you'll be surprised at the marvelous effects you can come up with.

Lighting and Sound

Be as selective as you can when choosing your lighting man or woman. Good lighting is very important in a fashion show. You need a good "spot" man who can turn on the right color. Put the wrong color on a costume and you can ruin the look of it. Give him a lineup sheet.

Sometimes you can't afford a professional lighting man or any kind of elaborate lighting setup. If you have to work with homemade apparatus and you have only a stationary light, a pink or white light would be best and safest.

Test your microphone before showtime. This is very important.

PRODUCING YOUR SHOW

Now that you know the basics of your behind-the-scenes planning, let's get to work on what will appear onstage. There are so many things that go into this phase of your planning. You'll have to decide on a theme, figure out the price range of the clothes you will show, choose your commentator, and the clothes she will talk about, and use actual stage techniques.

Selecting a Theme

A fashion-show theme can be built around a season, or an occasion, or the type of women who will be viewing the production. It should be brief and have a definite meaning.

The group that is giving the fashion show should look for key words that are currently being used in the fashion world. You might possibly build your title around this word. For instance, last year they were using "Happening." They're still using it. You can work this into a catchy title in many different ways.

Start out with a simple "Fashion Happening" or "Springtime Happening," but word it in such a way that you can build and be as original as you like within a short title. I think it's the clever little touches that make all the difference.

Of course, the commentary will have to be built around this theme up to a point, but don't be afraid to be original. Make up something more imaginative than just "Springtime Fashions" or "Fall Fashions." You can do better than that!

Your Script

Use scenes to give your fashion show meaning. You can have four, six, eight scenes. You may have as many as you think you can handle, within reason.

Let's assume you have six scenes. Your opening scene would be "Sports." "Daytime" would be second, "Travel," third, "Theatre," fourth, "Cocktail Party," fifth, and "Formal," sixth.

This can vary in many ways. It might be a "Swimming Party" and you'll show a whole scene of bathing suits, or "Outdoor Fun" and you'll build it around several outdoor sports.

Build your own scenes, even if the subject is a housewife—in the kitchen, on the patio, or gardening. What will she wear gardening? You can have many brief scenes, but I don't want to complicate it too much. I'm just suggesting how to put on a fashion show for an organization, and I'm not trying—much as I would like to!—to make a big production of it.

In an opening scene, since all the models are dressed, it's really very effective to have most of them onstage when the curtain opens. You may position them around the setting or in a group. Let them model, one at a time, or two at a time. Whichever you like. This makes a marvelous grand opening.

From then on, the models will need time to dress. With an organization—where the girls aren't professionals who are able to dress quickly—eight or ten models would be used. Ten would be best, because then they would have plenty of time to change. With professionals, you can do it with six models. They can dress quickly. Eight is certainly much easier. I wish I could always use eight in a fashion show, but organizations can't always afford eight professionals, so six are used. Eight or ten are ideal.

If an organization would like to have more of their members model, there is nothing wrong with having sixteen models, if they choose, and have fewer changes. Instead of wearing six changes, let each model wear four or even three so that all can have a chance to participate.

Have a theme and have different scenes. If you have enough models, they can come out in different groups or colors.

The Price Range of Your Clothes

Key the price range of your fashion show to the type of women who are attending, but don't be afraid to go into a few extravagant items. Do show a few sheer luxury items because women like to see them. They like to splurge a little. On the other hand, you do want the store to sell clothes. That's the object of any store even wanting to participate in your showing and going to the trouble of presenting its fashions. Stores hope to make some sales, so keep the prices within the reach of your audience.

In mentioning price, it's good to have a variety of prices in a fashion show, to showcase what the store has, unless it's a tremendously exclusive shop that has only very expensive clothes. Perhaps your audience will consist mainly of the type of woman who would be interested in an exclusive shop. It's up to the women in your organization to figure out the type of person you hope — or are able — to attract.

Please the audience with the price range, but make it a little flexible. In one of my shows, for instance, I had prices ranging from $50 to $350. A woman may not be able to afford more than a $50 garment, so she should find at least some things she can buy. A woman who would prefer something more expensive would have her choice of clothes that cost up to $350.

Prices can be much less. Simply make them suitable to your audience, and always go a little higher on some items.

Types of Models

Naturally, you'll select your models from members of the club, their families, and possibly volunteers from your community. If you choose your types from a Petite up to a Matron model, you'll have a much happier audience. You might, of course, be planning to direct your fashion show to a young and swinging audience. In that case, go all out with High Fashion and Junior models.

Ordinarily, however, you should try to adapt your types and sizes to a wider range. I hesitate to have a size 22. I've tried it, and it hasn't gone over very well. Avoid going over a size 16 in a fashion show. Women who are very large have a reluctance to see themselves in that category. They know that they certainly can dress — and look — better. This, again, is up to the group giving the show. If you think you can do it successfully, go ahead.

In general, I would recommend: Children, Petites, and up to size 16. Make it an interesting show and a varied one — and gear it to the needs of the women in your community.

Makeup for Your Models

There are several ways you can handle this. One is for the models themselves to apply their own makeup, using what they've learned from the makeup chapter in this book. Another way would be for you to have one or two girls — members of your organization or volunteer friends — who are proficient in the art assist the girls who aren't too skillful. A third way would make use of professional help, in exchange for publicity for their assistance.

You might ask one of your local cosmetic firms, shops, or boutiques to come backstage and assist with the makeup, and put finishing touches to it. In return for this, they may put their samples on your tables. You can also give them publicity or advertising in your program and in the fashion show itself.

Such firms are usually very willing to cooperate if they're going to get free publicity, and they will most likely donate some time to the show. At least, it's worth a try. We've done it with some of our shows, then talked about their makeup, and let them put their brochures on the tables.

You could do this, too, with a local hairdresser or wig shop, if you like, depending on how elaborate you intend your production to be, and how handy your girls are with their hair.

The Role of the Commentator

Your commentator is a key figure in your fashion show. Choose her carefully, as she can either make your show a bright and lively production or turn it into a dull and plodding exercise. Of course, you'll have the clothes to liven things up, but it's up to your commentator to integrate the entire performance and make it a smooth and cohesive whole.

You will have to select a woman who is versatile. She will have to put her commentary together, analyze the fashions so that she can discuss them intelligently, and she must have a pleasant speaking voice. Also very much needed are an unshakable poise and the ability to ad-lib if the occasion demands it. Be sure you choose a woman who has clear diction as well as a beautifully modulated voice, someone who finds it easy to speak and doesn't have stage fright.

If you were the commentator, this is the way you would work. Fittings will normally be one or two days ahead. In a fashion show with experienced help, the fittings can be the day before. Two days before, at the most, because the stores wouldn't want their merchandise out of the departments longer than that.

Let's say the show is slated for a Saturday. The fittings would be on Thursday, starting early in the morning. Allow an hour for fittings for each model, depending on how much help there is in the store. Sometimes you can have two girls go in at one time in an hour, but don't have them all gang up at the shop — half a dozen at a time — unless the store can accommodate such a number.

If you want them all there at one time, it might be possible to have fittings after the store closes. If this can be arranged, fine. Have several salesgirls stay over, and they can each take two girls. Knowing the lineup of the show, then you can see everything lined up at one time. Otherwise, send the girls in one at a time, an hour apart, throughout the day.

At the fittings, each model will fill out slips of paper, listing the numbers and descriptions of the costumes she's wearing. You will take them from her, and work out your general commentary from them. (See example of such a slip on page 237.) There are six costumes in this case, but it could be any number. You will look over the clothes, and the general information is there. You can add little bits yourself. You will see the clothes and recognize them in your mind when you go home to write up your cards.

With an inexperienced commentator, sometimes even with an experienced one, emphasis should be placed on the importance of writing a card. One card for each garment, and cards will be numbered in the order in which the models come out. There are eight models wearing six changes—six times eight is forty-eight—so there will be forty-eight cards numbered that way. Professionals have various ways to prepare their commentaries; however, you will find this best for you.

Put the girl's name up in the lefthand corner, typing it in capitals so that it's easy to read, and the number in the center. Always start the card with the "Opening," to set the scene, so to speak. If your model is wearing a bathing suit, it could read something like this:

"Mary will enjoy a day at the beach, while she looks delightful in her cool, green nylon two-piece suit from (store's name)."

Here are samples of two ways a model can fill out information for the coordinator after she has had her fittings. Decide which way you want your models to follow. I would suggest you do a sample card for the girls to see. This will help you receive the information from them more accurately.

Sample of Card Model Gives to Coordinator

PAULINE SULLIVAN   RONZONES

1. Green pant dress, front zip, blue pockets, blue flower on zipper. Cotton and dacron. $25.00
2. Brown wool knit, white trim, A-shape, lined. $50.00
3. Black-and-white houndstooth, 2-piece sleeveless dress and jacket. Wool blend. Fully lined. $70.00
4. Pink crepe short cocktail dress, trimmed with orange and pink ostrich feathers at hemline, lined. $95.00
Location: In the Boulevard Shopping Center. Maryland Parkway and Desert Inn Road.

No.	Scene & Name	Color	Fabric	Design	Designer	Accessories	Detail Description
1	*Sports* Capri Set	Turq. blue	Wool knit	2-piece	Roxanne	Brown leather boots, white felt beret.	Zip jacket, patch pock., bell leg. $49.95
2	*Daytime* Wool Dress	Red	Mohair & wool	1-piece, A-shape	Mr. Mort	Navy shoes & bag, leather, navy gloves, red & navy hat.	Lined dress, pleats, stitched bodice. $50.00
3	*Travel* Suit	Black-&-white tweed	Wool & linen	3-piece	Mandlyn	Black leather shoes & bag, white gloves.	Sleeveless shell, cardigan jacket. $95.00
4	*Theatre* Costume Ensemble	Hot pink	Silk lined	A-shape, Empire	Trigère	Pink silk shoes, beige leather bag & gloves.	Jewel but., same fabr., piping-lined bow at back. $350.00
5	*Cocktail* Party Dress	Black	Silk shantung	1-Piece, sheath	Ozzie	Black silk shoes, black silk eve. bag; sht. blk. kid gloves.	Ostrich feather hemline. $90.00
6	*Formal* Party Long Evening	White	Crepe	1-piece Princess	Larry	White silk shoes, white beaded bag; wht. gl., fox cape.	Rhine. trim & pearls, lined & interlined. $250.00

This form can be mimeographed easily. Models simply fill in information.

Take each model's information, and as you look at the clothes check the card for information. Add anything extra you may desire. You will have something to work with for your commentary if you plan to write it out more elaborately.

Go ahead and talk about the fit of it, the cut of it, the line of it, the fabric. Make your comments as if you were talking and selling the bathing suit. Remember, a commentator is an asset to a show. You should talk in a warm tone, clearly and distinctly and not too rapidly. You can hesitate occasionally and let the models simply walk for a moment, focusing attention on the accessories that a model might be wearing from the different accessory departments. If they are the girl's own accessories, naturally you would not comment on them.

It is important that a commentator learn not to be monotonous in her tone. Be enthusiastic. Feel enthusiasm. Your voice must show it. You should talk quickly sometimes, sometimes slowly, sometimes seriously, sometimes intimately. This is why I keep reemphasizing the need for a woman who speaks beautifully and who won't freeze with stage fright. Even if you're reading the cards, don't sound as if you're reading them.

If you have a large enough card, you can double-space your information. Actually, double-spacing is easier for some women, though I manage quite nicely with single spacing. Have all your cards the same size; 4 inches by 6 inches is fairly standard. You can get larger ones if you like. You can get more information on them, and you may not have to turn the card over.

As you write out your cards, you really are giving yourself a review, and it will be helpful if you can go off and do this by yourself. You should have a list of adjectives and expressions that are used in describing clothes. You can select these from fashion magazines and from fashion columns in the newspapers. They will be of tremendous value in helping you to characterize something that's new for the season. Generally the coordinator is also the commentator, but this wouldn't necessarily be so. Some groups may put on a fashion show with a director, and also enlist a commentator who may work with the coordinator.

If you're going to have someone else write your descriptions, someone who is clever with words, you should have the cards far enough in advance to enable you to read them over and over and become familiar with the wording on them. You must be comfortable with the words and they mustn't appear "new" to you.

Have one of your group's members check to see that the music doesn't drown out your voice. Place your microphone on the opposite side of the stage from the music. The music should be on one side; the commentator on the other. At least you should be far enough away from the music so that you will be clearly heard.

You should have a copy of the lineup of the show. Besides your separate cards, you will have a complete list of the lineup in front of you so that you can glance at it quickly. (See the example shown on page 237.) In case a card should slip out of sight or something unexpected happens—such as a model coming out at the wrong time! —you will have that list and notice quickly that Mary's onstage instead of Jane. Then you quickly find Mary's card with the description of her costumes and, seeing that she's in an unscheduled dress, you ad-lib.

Incidentally, these model sheets for the separate fittings of the girls are excellent to give each girl, so that she'll know the lineup of her own clothes, and know the accessories she'll have to wear.

Should you talk about prices? Yes. Women do like to hear about prices. In more and more fashion shows, prices are quoted. It's only when you get into extremely expensive items that prices are not quoted. Ask any woman. She likes to hear the price, and I'd suggest you mention it.

Be original when describing your scenes. Don't just say, "Sports," "Theatre," "Evening," and so on. These are basically what will be shown, but you can give them more exciting titles—on your program, too—and call them something like "On the Riviera," or "Our First Trip to Europe," or "First Stop—Acapulco." Anything like that, or whatever you want to come up with. Let your imagination go and get yourself an exciting title for each scene.

Watch your fashion pages and see what other people are doing, and try to do better. You simply get your ideas from what's going on in the world around you. There are young people in the world, and they do exciting things. Build your show around your community and the things it does. You can build it around travel and vacations, or around brides. A bridal scene is always a showstopper. Some seasonal collections are climaxed with a big dramatic bridal tableau. You can take it a bit farther and show a whole bridal wardrobe and all the things a bride would be wearing on her honeymoon.

Coming back to your commentary, if you are a novice and this is your first appearance in this capacity, it might help if you have a word-for-word script of what you're going to say. After you become proficient at it, you can say, "I don't need this. I have key words and I have a list of them in front of me." In the beginning, learn to almost memorize certain ways of describing things. Eventually, they become second nature to you; such phrases as "Lace cascading down the front and around the neckline . . ."

There are many different ways to delineate a fashion, and you learn from reading the fashion pages. They will come to the tip of your tongue with the aid of little key words, which is the way I do my own commentaries. I wouldn't advise a girl just coming in and doing a show for the first time to do it this way. You should really *look* at the costume, and not repeat monotonous phrases or the same adjectives or descriptive words.

Another important thing to remember is that even though you read your commentary—which, as a newcomer, you will have to do— you must become so familiar with the words that it doesn't seem as if you are reading. For example, here is a description that is written out completely:

"Another facet of fashion is the dazzler for hostess wear. It's Open House at Lillian's and she's not worrying about what to serve, for all eyes will feast on how marvelous she looks in black-sequined Capris, topped with white chiffon and a black chiffon overskirt. Any woman will certainly feel great looking like this. It is completely lined with silk and truly has a look of distinction. The price: $110."

Unfortunately, when you read a card, it sounds like reading. This is why I very much dislike writing out much more than an opening. I look at a garment and I can see what it's like. It's much better this way. I'm looking at a magazine, and if I were describing the girl I'm looking at right now, I would say it this way:

"Another facet of fashion is the dazzler for hostess wear. It's Open House at Lillian's, but she isn't worried at all about what to serve, for she's going to be the center of attention, as everyone looks at this perfectly beautiful black-sequined Capri. It's all topped with very feminine white chiffon, and isn't the black chiffon overskirt most exciting? A woman will look forward to having guests when she's wearing this. Its price? $110. And she'll enjoy it for many, many months— enjoy always feeling that luxurious touch of chiffon."

Do you see the difference? See how much better and more spontaneous the second version is than the first? The first one is good enough, but you don't want that. You want something better. Don't sound stilted. Become so familiar with the card that you can take your eyes off it and look at the garment being modeled.

Look at the sample card the model gives to the coordinator (on page 236). You may take the information just as it is on the card and add it below your opening sentence. Or you may take the information and write it out word for word, as our sample card shows below. We will take the first costume the model was to wear. One card for each costume, remember!

SAMPLE COMMENTARY CARD

PAULINE SULLIVAN   I   RONZONES

FOR YOU WOMEN WHO WANT FREEDOM OF LEG MOVEMENT AND THE LOOK OF A SKIRT ... THE PANT DRESS IS YOUR ANSWER. HERE IS A NEW SHADE OF GREEN FOR SPRING ... CELERY GREEN. ... IT LOOKS SO COOL, AND THE MARVELOUS BLUE ACCENT OF THE PATCH POCKET ALONG WITH THE FUN LITTLE FLOWER ATTACHED TO THE ZIPPER CLOSING. JUST A WHISK OF THE IRON IS ALL THAT WILL BE NEEDED FOR THIS WASHABLE BLEND OF COTTON AND DACRON ... $25.00

As you become more professional you can work from the card as the model gives it to you.

You won't remember everything—for some reason—unless it's written down. *Write everything down.* If you're supposed to have a little break in the middle of the show, either for a spot of entertainment or to proceed with a raffle, write it on a card and place the card in the middle of the pack. It will follow the last number before the break, so that when you see it you'll know that this is the time to do it. A closing card of thanks is important also.

Staging Your Fashion Show

Once the commentator has been introduced, and this introduction should be written down so that your chairman will know exactly what to say, the show can go on. A word about introductions. Keep them short and sweet and flattering. If the fashion show can go on undisturbed, it will have more continuity and beauty about it. It should be a smooth production from beginning to end, and the first steps to your shining success will be the rehearsals.

REHEARSALS

Allow sufficient rehearsal time for the girls who are learning from this book. If it will make them feel better, schedule a couple of rehearsals, but you must have at least one. The best way is to have a rehearsal at someone's house to work out ideas, and then a full rehearsal on the actual stage or area you'll be using. Let the girls become

accustomed to the place from which they're expected to make an entrance, and give them the feel of the room. This will be of tremendous
help.

Get your girls to move. You have to learn to give orders, and they'll
follow them. If you stand around, not saying anything, they'll do the
same. Children in the fashion show should be at rehearsal, too. They
should know the feel of the room, where they're going to dress, how
they're going to enter. Practice your opening and your finale. If you're
going to work any groups together, or colors, these, of course, should
be rehearsed.

Let's say that you're the coordinator. You can do many different
things with fashions. You can have two or three models come out in
the same color tones. One will model, and then the other. Sometimes
you will have them model together up to a certain point and then separate. Or they can model together, then one will go to one side of the
stage, and one, to the other. As you see more production fashion shows,
you will gather ideas. You can let your imagination run wild, but when
you're working on a production you have to have an idea of what you're
doing, and don't be afraid to try it. It may not work in actual practice,
but you won't know until you try it. (Review Chapter 6 on "Group
Modeling.")

STAGING THE SCENES

As long as each girl has time to dress, whether you have eight
models or more, let each follow the same girl throughout the show.
Each model will receive a number; for eight models you would have
Numbers 1 through 8. You'll know that when Model No. 1 is showing,
Model No. 2 should be ready or onstage with her, possibly even Model
No. 3. The other girls should be dressing. Follow an even-paced routine. You would not take Model No. 1 and slip her into fifth position.
Sometimes this can be done in the last part of the show, or when you
want to squeeze a girl in, if she can dress that rapidly. You should try
to work your girls with the same numbers throughout. Professional
models dress more rapidly and can be changed around, but I do not
advise this with beginners.

TIMING

Usually you can figure that a model will take about a minute on
a fairly large stage, but bring a stopwatch with you to rehearsal and
find out for yourself how long a model stays onstage or on the runway.
Clock it. If you have eight or ten models, let them go through their
paces on the runway and clock how long it takes for the whole group.

Then if you have six changes for each model, six times that is ap-

proximately how long your fashion show will last. If it took ten minutes for ten models, who showed six garments each, your time would
be sixty minutes. That's on a full stage, one model at a time. A minute
is a little long, possibly. Thirty-six costumes shouldn't take longer
than thirty-six minutes. Eight models would take forty-eight minutes.

The time required would depend on how your girls are paced.
They shouldn't walk too slowly; there should be a fairly brisk pace
to make it exciting. If a girl drags it out, or stays on too long, it becomes
monotonous. By all means, she should stay onstage long enough so
that everyone in the room can see what she is wearing. This is where
rehearsals will be so helpful, as they also will be in letting you follow
the runway and stage formats which you've learned in this book.

The models will learn that backstage they have to dress quickly
and have all their clothes lined up properly. Backstage organization
is vital. As soon as a girl is offstage, she starts undressing. There's
no time for conversation or for anything other than preparing for the
next outfit. Here is where your lineup sheet will aid your models so
that they'll know exactly where they're supposed to be.

A lineup sheet consists of the models' names in the order of modeling. Each model will have a number, and thus she can see who pre-
cedes her as well as who follows. The lineup sheet may or may not show
the costumes each model will be wearing. (This is discussed below.)
Often, extra charts are made for "Openings" and "Finales," to avoid
any mistakes.

THE LINEUP SHEET

There are several ways to set up a lineup sheet. I'll show you two
of them, with samples and illustrations. For examples, we will use
Sample Lineup Sheet No. 1, using eight models, and Sample Lineup
Sheet No. 2, which we followed for the American Business Women's
Association, using models in group scenes.

Explanation of Lineup Sheet No. 1

Take a sheet of regular typwriting paper, and using a ruler 1 inch
wide, start 1 inch from the top and square the sheet off in 1-inch blocks.
The previous line made by the ruler is the line you follow. You may
use carbons to save time. One page will be sufficient for the model's
name and the six changes she will wear. If there are more changes
in the show, simply attach another squared-off page to this one with
Scotch tape. If there are more models, do the same at the bottom of
the first sheet you have made. Use the plain, top-inch border for the
name of the fashion show, who it is for, place, date, and time. Also,
list the scene names above each square.

Each model can see what number she occupies in the lineup and what outfit she wears in each scene. Looking down the page, you can see at a glance what costumes will be worn in the sports scene and in each scene that follows. Looking across the page, the model can see how her clothes should be lined up in the order she is to wear them. Color and type of costume are all that are necessary. The commentator's cards will have the full description of each costume. The models may or may not have a personal chart made out. This will be up to the coordinator, or the model may do this herself. The lineup sheet is very important for the lighting man and the musician to see what scenes and colors follow each model.

SAMPLE LINEUP SHEET NO. 1

FASHION SHOW FOR _____ DATE _____
PLACE _____ TIME _____

NAME	SPORTS	TRAVEL	RELAXING	DAYTIME	AFTER FIVE	FORMAL
1. YVONNE MONGEON	White military pantsuit	Orange knit, 3-piece	Print knit p.j.'s	Red knit separates	Black chiffon	White crepe rhinestone
2. PAULINE SULLIVAN	Pink Capri's	Yellow knit 2-piece suit	Brown hostess dress	Navy knit dress	White crepe	Green brocade
3. RUTH LESLIE	Knit green mini dress	Biege & brown wool suit	Navy knit p.j.'s	White wool coat dress	Royal blue silk	Blue crepe
4. CAROL STEELE	Print nylon bathing suit	Coat & dress, pink wool knit	Red Capri set, wool	Purple knit suit	White and gold	Black silk
5. JILL DIEHL	Yellow & white cotton dress	Black & white 3-piece suit	Hawaiian print, cotton	Gray wool dress	Powder blue wool & silk	Pink pearl trim
6. CHERYL REESE	Bathing suit, 2-piece	Brown & white cotton suit	Polka dot navy & white pant dress	Black wool, white trim	Yellow & white silk beaded	Beige & brown
7. JUANITA CHEEK	Black & white pantsuit	Red knit dress & coat	Black & white shift, long	Hot pink dress	Silver & white	Black & white
8. JUDI MOREO	Blue pant dress	Blue & red coat dress	Orange & pink print cotton, long dress	Green print dress	Beige & fur trim	Yellow silk

Note: Even numbers Stage Right, odd numbers Stage Left

We will use the first model, Yvonne Mongeon, as an example of a personal chart she would make up for herself.

Explanation of Lineup Sheet No. 2

We did this show for an audience of three thousand women, and we kept each scene in a special color. Because there were so many models, I gave them all numbers from 1 through 5, and divided them into five groups.

Group 1 had five models, Group 2 had four, Group 3 had five, Group 4 had four, and Group 5 had five. There were five models in almost every group except the children's. As each scene carried out a color, it wasn't important for the girls to know the fabric or anything else. They just had to remember that in the first scene all of them were in stripes. In the second scene, they wore navy and yellow; in the third, was black and white, and in the fourth, silver and gold for evening. They modeled on an 80-foot runway.

Looking at Lineup Sheet No. 2, you can see that each scene was done by a whole group. In Lineup Sheet No. 1, each model's costume is listed separately by color and style, and would be so shown, unless a note were added that two or more models were to make an appearance onstage at the same time. In Lineup No. 1, each girl modeled alone. Just be certain that there is enough time for the models to dress between each change.

SAMPLE LINEUP SHEET NO. 2

AMERICAN BUSINESS WOMEN'S ASSOCIATION FASHION SHOW

PLACE   THEME   DATE

(Keep each scene in a special color, fabric, theme.)

NAME	SCENE 1	SCENE 2	SCENE 3	SCENE 4
1. FRAN ZALATEL 2. SANDRA WALKER 3. JUDY MATHIS 4. PAT MC COWN 5. JEALETTA	COLOR Stripes mini	Navy & yellow	Black & white	Silver & gold Evening
1. LORI STARDEVANT 2. JEANNETTE CAJA 3. BETTY OAKES 4. SHARON ROCK	Green & orange	Hostess	Furs	Color Short evening
1. MARY ALLEN 2. JANET BRUCE 3. CAROL STEEL 4. VALERIE BARNES 5. BETTY BRIAN	Coordinates Capris & skirts gold & brown	Pantsuits	Green, gold, orange	Long formals
1. TOBI SALTZMAN 2. BRIGETTE BILRAY 3. KELLY DUKE 4. CHARLOTTE CALUNGA CHILDREN	Daytime red, white & blue	Coats	Party	Wait for Finale
1. CAROL NEY 2. JOAN WICKMAN 3. WILMA FERDINAND 4. DALE SMITH 5. IRENE BAILEY	Daytime blue with other color	Navy & red	Furs	Black & white evening

---

Lineup Sheets—Where, How, and Who

A lineup sheet should be posted in the dressing room where it is most convenient for all the models to see. You should possibly have two of them, with one near the doorway where models can check it as they go out. Sometimes a stage manager (or stagehand) will have one in hand. If you possibly can, make six or seven copies, two for the models' room; if there are men, one for their dressing room; one for the lighting man so that he'll know what color will be shown in each scene; one for the musician; and one for the stage manager and assistant coordinator.

The responsibility of the assistant coordinator is to see that the models get out on time and in the proper order. She will be standing in the wings.

Anyone who needs a lineup sheet should have one. The commentator has one, of course, but she also will have more elaborate information on cards.

If You Have More Scenes

If each model is showing eight or ten garments, rather than six, another piece of paper should be used. You don't have to mark the model's name again. Just attach the second piece of paper to the side of the first one with Scotch tape. Use average 8 by 11 paper, and add your changes in the proper order.

Insert a little note at the bottom of the sheet, reminding your models that they will be coming out in group settings, that they should smile, and keep moving. Anything the director might want to add could be inserted here also. On No. 1, we noted that even-numbered models were to come out on Stage Right and odd-numbered ones on Stage Left.

Any information should be typed for the models. Not only do you tell them, but with written material, you'll be less apt to make mistakes.

OPENINGS AND FINALES

All of your fashion show should be beautiful, but you want your opening and finale to be absolutely smashing. Get your show off to a brilliant start, and end it in a burst of glory. (Study "Finales" in Chapter 6.)

Here are some general pointers on openings and finales.

Openings

A word of caution. For an opening scene with all your models on-stage, you may want them spaced differently than in the order of their numbers. Remembering to allow time for the models to dress, each one should follow the same number as on the lineup sheet. With six or eight models, this is almost a must.

Example: Visualize six models onstage. You want them to model one at a time and then go offstage. We're showing you the right way and the wrong way to stage this evenly:

I	II
Not this	*This is better*
1 2 3 4 5 6	1 3 5 6 4 2

In II, each girl steps forward and models according to her number in the lineup. After Model No. 1 finishes and goes off, Model No. 2 follows, and so on. When Model No. 6 has finished, Model No. 1 will be dressed and ready to be onstage.

Finales

Bear in mind the coloring and heights of the models for the finales. You may want to space the models in various groups rather than in a half-circle or a straight line across the stage. Have fun with your stage and props. The models are all through with the show, so the props can now be moved on the stage to where they will be most effective.

If possible, it is much more effective to let a curtain close with your models onstage. However, if this is impossible, have them practice walking offstage attractively. Half can go one way, and half can go the other. The models may go off on one side, or cross over for another exit idea. Just be sure that a model knows she is the one to lead the rest offstage. Remind all the models to keep an even distance and to keep moving.

You can refer back to any of the eight stage and runway finales that we've outlined in Chapter 6. However you want your models to go off, give the explanation and draw the diagram. Again, don't forget to indicate on the diagram the name of the model who is to lead the others off. Explain every detail. This will be very helpful to the model.

Remind your models that they won't always get these diagrams, but as we're offering suggestions on how to give a fashion show with nonprofessionals, we want to make it easy and meaningful for them. Even with professionals, it is a good idea to do this. It will ensure that the girls understand and won't be able to say, "Oh, you didn't tell me!" It's right there in black and white. Nothing is more appalling for a coordinator or a director than to have a model alibi a mishap with the "you-didn't-tell-me" routine. If you've written it down, there it is.

Last-Minute Checkup

We've brought you straight through a fashion show from its inception in your mind to the diagram for your rousing — we hope — finale. You're ready for the big day. Don't forget those last-minute — and in some cases, not-so-last-minute — checkups.

It's very important for the coordinator and the commentator to check everything carefully the day before to make sure that each task necessary for the show has been accomplished. The programs must be made up and ready, and you should know who's going to deliver them. Your hostesses, or your ushers, if you're having them, should be ready for duty. If there are any souvenirs to be given out, are all the little gifts ready for the tables? Have there been any changes in casting, or name changes of *any* kind? Make sure the new name is included, even if it has to be written in. They do it in Broadway shows, so you can do it.

Does the dress shop know where to deliver the clothes? Don't laugh — clothes have been delivered to the wrong place before! Does the shop know the clothes have to be there at least an hour before showing, and do you have someone backstage to protect them?

Check dressing-room facilities with the management of the locale of your fashion show, whether it's a hotel room, clubroom, or dining room. Wherever the models are dressing, they will need mirrors and a clothes rack. Possibly the dress shop may supply these. Usually, a hotel will have them. Make sure that each model has a place to put her hatbox and a place to sit.

An hour before show time, be sure to check your microphone, your lights, and any props that should be in place. If there's a change of scenery, who does this? Be sure the persons responsible are backstage and know their cues.

All of these things must go smoothly and must be double-checked. Do your wardrobe women know which models they're dressing? Are your lineup sheets taped up on the wall? Does everyone who should have a lineup sheet have one? This includes your lighting man, musician, and stage manager.

Your chairman should have her little speech of introduction written out. Make it short and to the point and exciting. Thanking people who have helped is fine, if it isn't too long a list. Sometimes it's best to mention them in the program and elaborate less verbally.

One thing I do like in a club endeavor like this is to include in the program the name of every woman who assisted in any way. This is appreciated and is a very nice gesture. You can have all your acknowledgments on the back of the program.

An important factor in the organization of fashion shows is to make each member proud to have been part of it. People like to be recognized. You might have everyone who participated in producing the fashion show stand, so that all will get a great hand. It would show the audience how many women were necessary to work to bring the show to them. Don't forget to thank the guests for attending your show, whether to help their favorite charity or some special group goal.

Thank the society editors and other members of the press.

I hope I've covered every aspect of putting on a fashion show. Having done so, there's really only one thing left to say: On with the show!

13
ROOM AT THE TOP!

There are top models and top agencies, and from their dizzying heights the elite of the industry can gaze down on their glamorous holdings with well-justified satisfaction. While it's not exactly crowded up there, there is—for the girl who is willing, ambitious, and properly equipped—still room at the top.

Following is a photographic gallery of models from various top model agencies throughout the United States.

Wilhelmina Cooper, formerly a top model for the Ford Model Agency, now heads her own Wilhelmina Model Agency, one of the leaders in the field.

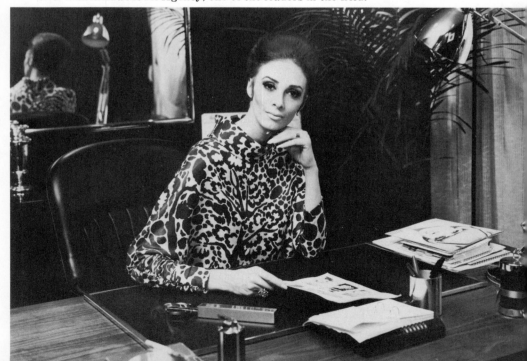

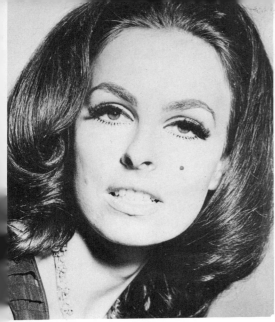

KARIN ALEXANA

Sabie Models, Inc., Chicago

Age: 21   Hair: Brown
Size: 8 - 10   Eyes: Brown
Height: 5 feet 8½ inches

Karin is a native of Germany and started her career in modeling during her teens there. Cosmetics and fashions have always fascinated her. Karin feels the best medicine for beauty is plenty of sleep, outdoor exercise such as ice skating, which she loves. She admits to working hard at always looking like a model and changing her appearance as fashion dictates and still maintain her own personality. Keeping an optimistic viewpoint is vital to a model, even if you have to fake it.

DEE ANNA

Plaza Three Model Agency, Phoenix, Arizona

Age: 26   Hair: Blonde
Size: 8   Eyes: Hazel
Height: 5 feet 8 inches

Dee Anna started as a teen model in Chicago. She has had experience in every type of fashion modeling, and feels that being versatile is very important in her work. Like many models, she has traveled —to the Orient, Europe, and Mexico. She likes being settled in Phoenix, where modeling is less hectic yet keeps her busy enough.

Photo by Robert B. Ross

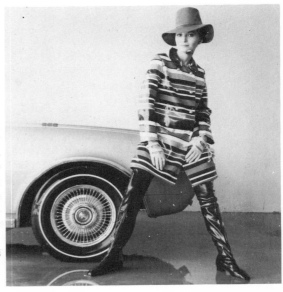

NANCY BENNETT

Shore Model Agency, Asbury Park, New Jersey

Age: Past 40   Hair: Silver
Size: 12 - 14   Eyes: Brown
Height: 5 feet 10 inches

Nancy has been modeling for over thirty years. She is a wife, and the mother of a twenty-one-year-old daughter and a fifteen-year-old son. She formerly modeled in New York for Hattie Carnegie, Pattullo, and Maurice Rentner. She enjoys combining her role as wife, mother, and model, and feels that being able to exude your own personality and to look genuine to your audience is of prime importance for a superior model.

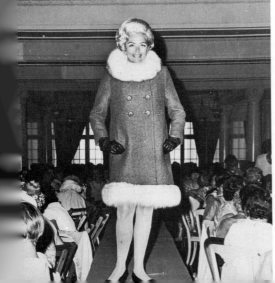

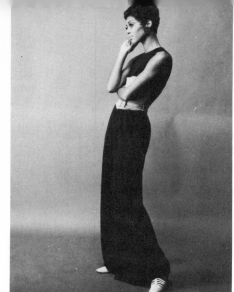

CARMEN

Wilhemina Model Agency, New York
Age: 23   Hair: Black
Size: 7-8   Eyes: Brown
Height: 5 feet 7½ inches

Carmen was born in Seattle, Washington, and began her modeling career by working as a stylist. She firmly believes each model should create her own individual look, and in copying a fashion trend always add her own unique ideas. Versatility is as important in appearance as ability is in modeling techniques. She loves the traveling and challenging excitement of modeling. Her travels have included Europe and the Middle East. She enjoys dancing and sewing in what spare time she can manage.

Photo by Larry Stewart

SHARLA CARTWRIGHT

Estelle Compton Models, Minneapolis, Minnesota
Age: 30   Hair: Brown
Size: 8   Eyes: Blue
Height: 5 feet 6 inches

Sharla was born in Sioux Falls, South Dakota. She started her modeling career in her late twenties. She is a former airline stewardess and placed first and second place in two airline beauty contests. It is still a surprise to her that she is so much in demand for fashion shows in her area. Sharla stays very busy maintaining a happy home and raising five children with her husband. Besides modeling she loves to paint and bowl and play tennis with her husband.

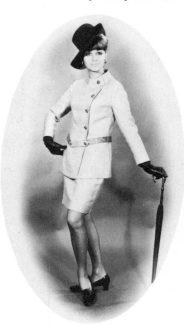

ANGELYN FORBES

Shore Model Agency, Asbury Park, New Jersey
Age range: 17-24   Hair: Brown
Size: 6-7-8   Eyes: Brown
Height: 5 feet 6 inches

Angelyn combines her modeling assignments with being a busy housewife. Her training and experience are extensive as you can read from our sample résumé on page 269. She feels that her experience as a wholesale model was invaluable, and would encourage other models to work at this before venturing into other modeling assignments. Her hobbies are gardening and decorating.

IRENE FREEMAN

Connecticut Model Agency, Inc., Stamford, Connecticut

Age: 45-55 Hair: Silver
Size: 12-14½ Eyes: Blue
Height: 5 feet 7½ inches

A versatile model, Irene is frequently seen in New York City and Connecticut department-store salon showings, and as the "Mother of the Bride." She has numerous television commercials to her credit. Her daughter Christie is a stunning 5 feet 9 inch-model with the same agency.

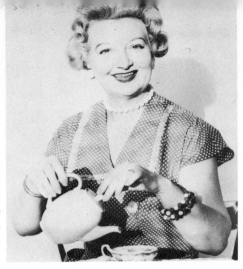

JANE HITCHCOCK

Wilhelmina Model Agency, New York

Age range: 15-23 Hair: Dark blonde
Size: 6-7-8 Eyes: Blue
Height: 5 feet 7 inches

A fifteen-year-old tycoon who lives with her mother and attends Manhattan's Professional Children's School, Jane grosses up to $600 a week, although her weekly allowance is $25, which covers her lunches, taxis, and school expenses.

Jane is from Vestavia, Alabama, and has always wanted to be a model. Under the direction of Wilhelmina, Jane has learned the fine art of makeup and photography modeling. Because of her great bone structure and versatility she is able to model teen fashions as well as more sophisticated assignments.

MONIKA JUST

Serendipity Talent Model Agency, New York

Age range: 18-23 Hair: Blonde
Size: 6-7-8 Eyes: Blue
Height: 5 feet 4 inches

Here is a perfect Petite or Junior model with marvelous bone structure. Monika photographs perfectly at any angle, and is used frequently for many different assignments in photography, commercials, and Junior size fashion modeling.

Photo by Richard Cassar

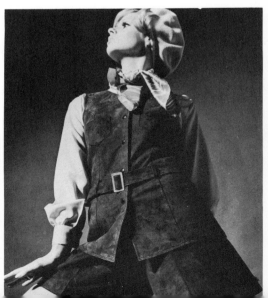

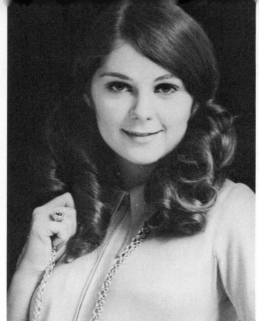

MARY BETH KLINE

Maezie Murphy Kline Model Agency, Palm Beach, Florida

Age: 20   Hair: Dark brown
Size: 8   Eyes: Brown
Height: 5 feet 7 inches

Mary Beth, who was born in Macon, Georgia, wants to continue modeling and study to be a teacher. She earns top money modeling for designers in Palm Beach and New York. You will see her in *Vogue*, *Glamour*, and *Mademoiselle* magazines. She's presently working for the famous designer Jacques Tiffeau in New York.

Photo by Philip E. Pegler

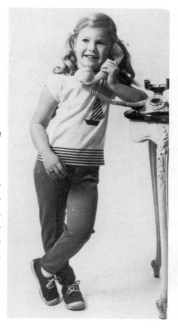

LISA KOENIG

Bonnie Kid Models Agency, New York
Age range: 5-6   Hair: Dark blonde
Size: 5-6   Eyes: Blue
Skin: Fair

Lisa is a very natural outgoing youngster who can relax in front of the camera and follow instructions with ease. She has learned at an early age that professionals cannot be known as temperamental. Do the job right is all important.

Photo by Al Belson

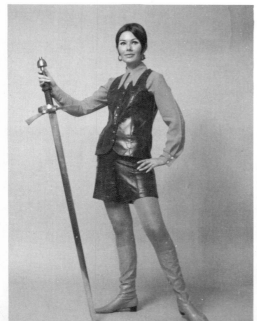

RUTH LESLIE

Lenz Model Agency, Las Vegas, Nevada
Age: 21   Hair: Red
Size: 8-10   Eyes: Green
Height: 5 feet 9 inches

Born in Hamburg, Germany, Ruth met and married an American serviceman and moved to Las Vegas. Bernie Lenz discovered her working in a dress shop and suggested that she train for modeling if she were interested. Ruth trained, and is now a top model working regularly in fashion shows, salons, and photography assignments. She plans to move to New York this year.

KIM LOCKWOOD

Lenz Model Agency, Las Vegas, Nevada
Age: 21 Hair: Blonde
Size: 7-8 Eyes: Blue
Height: 5 feet 8½ inches

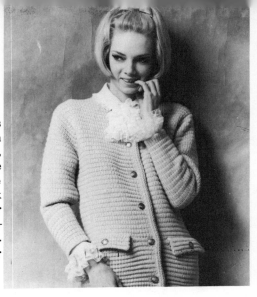

Kim has been modeling since she was sixteen years old. Although she is both a runway model and a photography model, Kim admits to being more comfortable in front of the camera. She was with the Wilhelmina Model Agency in New York for a short time, but likes the warmer West better. Her hobbies are designing clothes for herself and her friends.

Photo by Philip E. Pegler

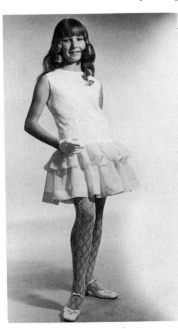

DONNA McGAUGHY

Lenz Model Agency, Las Vegas, Nevada
Age range: 10-14
Size: Child 14 and Pre-Teen 6-7-8
Height: 5 feet Eyes: Blue
Hair: Blonde

Donna has been studying ballet, tap, and acrobatics since the age of three. Her modeling career started after her training at the age of eight. She has modeled for many well-known designers of children's fashions both in stage, runway and tearoom fashion shows. One of her big thrills was her first visit to New York, where she modeled in the Waldorf Astoria Hotel. Her future plans are to continue more training in all the arts.

Photo by Al Belson

KITTY MEURLOTT

Plaza Three Model Agency, Phoenix, Arizona
Age: 55 Hair: Silver
Size: 12-14 Eyes: Blue
Height: 5 feet 7½ inches

Born in Montreal, Canada, Kitty moved to Phoenix, Arizona, when a small child. She enjoys modeling in between being a housewife and mother to four children ranging in ages from seventeen to twenty-two years. Swimming, knitting, and cooking are her hobbies. Kitty feels modeling has kept her alert to physical fitness and fashion awareness. She has traveled to Europe and Hawaii.

Photo by Robert B. Ross

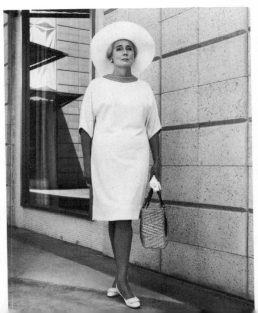

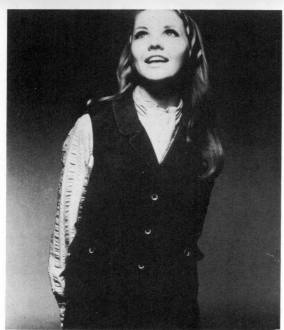

CAROL PHILLIPS

Wilhelmina Model Agency, New York
Age range: 18 - 24   Hair: Blonde
Size: 7 - 8   Eyes: Blue
Height: 5 feet 7½ inches

After training and modeling with the Lenz Model Agency in Nevada, Carol was selected to be a contestant in the "Professional Model Pageant," held at the Modeling Association of America Convention at the Waldorf Astoria Hotel, in 1968. Competing with 50 contestants from the states, Carol won first place and within a month was working through the Wilhelmina Model Agency in New York. She has been able to combine part-time nursing and part-time modeling, but admits it takes tremendous discipline.

CINDY PHILLIPS

Charm Associates Model Agency, Norfolk, Virginia
Age: 18   Hair: Brown
Size: 8 - 10   Eyes: Brown
Height: 5 feet 10 inches

Cindy is trying to do everything she desires at one time. At the moment she is attending Old Dominion College in Norfolk. Besides being a professional model, she is kept busy with promotion, fashion shows, and photography assignments. This picture was taken on a recent photography assignment in Florida.

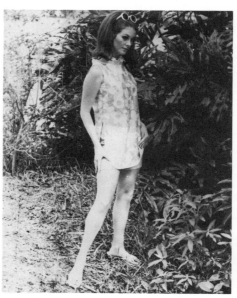

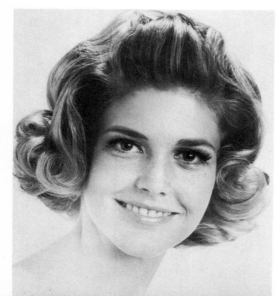

ANN STUART PICKETT

Maezie Murphy Kline Model Agency, Palm Beach, Florida
Age: 19   Hair: Frosted brown
Size: 8   Eyes: Hazel
Height: 5 feet 7 inches

Born in Bethesda, Maryland, Ann attends Palm Beach Junior College where she is studying retailing. Her hobbies are water skiing and teaching modeling at the agency where she is registered. She models for top designers and is the current "Ultra Brite Girl" with a $15,000 contract doing television commercials and public appearances.

SUSAN RATNER

Lenz Model Agency, Las Vegas, Nevada
Age: 21   Hair: Brown
Size: 7-8   Eyes: Brown
Height: 5 feet 8 inches

Susan will readily admit it took a great deal of training and experience for her to feel professional in modeling. Braces were needed to straighten her teeth during her teens. She trained and worked as a top Lenz fashion model in her teens, and has since modeled in New York, Los Angeles, and Phoenix. Susan says that part of the fun in modeling is the constant change one must make in appearance. There is always something new to look forward to in fashion. At the moment she is employed as an airline stewardess, and modeling part-time in Las Vegas.

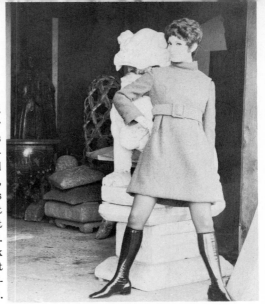

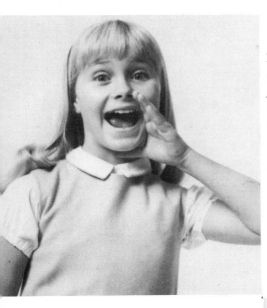

HEIDI ROOK

Bonnie Kid Models Agency, New York
Age range: 8-10   Hair: Dark blonde
Size: 8-10   Eyes: Blue
Skin: Fair

A very talented and hard-working child model, Heidi was selected to be featured in a Walt Disney film. You have seen her in catalogs, magazines, New York fashion shows, and television commercials. She dances, rides, models, and acts with ease. Like all professionals, she continually studies in all of these subjects.

TONYA SHOWALTER

House of Charm, San Francisco, California
Age range: 16-21   Hair: Blonde
Size: 8   Eyes: Brown
Height: 5 feet 7 inches

Living in this fascinating city and modeling there is a dream come true for Tonya. She has worked hard to be a good model. Loves to dress with a total look, and has found the majority of models exceptionally fine people. Her ambitions are to continue modeling, with a side interest in art. Tonya is seen often in the San Francisco fashion shows and Macy's ads.

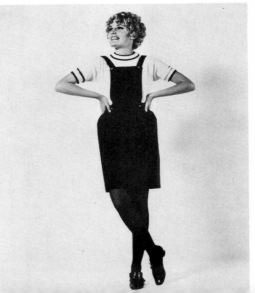

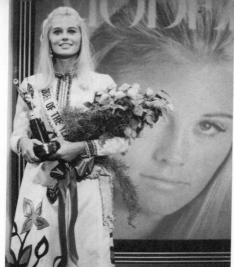

CYBILL SHEPHARD

Stewart Model Agency, New York
Age: 20   Hair: Blonde
Size: 8   Eyes: Blue
Height: 5 feet 8½ inches

1968 was a most thrilling year for Cybill —she won the "Model of the Year" contest. This annual pageant is produced by Stewart Model Agency and televised nationally. Cybill was on three magazine covers the first week and flew to Germany to do a commercial. With her solid bookings she is certain to earn more than her first-prize guarantee of $25,000. Memphis State University can be proud of this local girl who has become one of our top models. Tennis and golf are her favorite sports, when she has the time.

FAY SINCLAIR

Bonnie Kid Models Agency, New York
Age range: 4 - 5 - 6   Hair: Black
Size: 4 - 5 - 6   Eyes: Brown
Skin: Black

It is easy to see that Fay has all the sparkle necessary for a child model. Most important, she can turn different expressions on and off as directed. Children are born with a certain amount of charm, but much credit must be given to their parents and to the people who train them. Fay has learned the important saying, "The world does not revolve around a child."

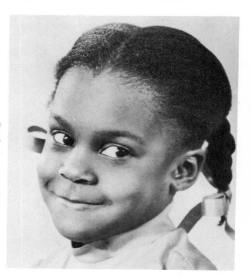

DOREE SOUTH

Alex Adams Model Agency, Louisville, Kentucky
Age: 19   Hair: Red
Size: 10 - 12   Eyes: Blue
Height: 5 feet 10 inches

Doree has been modeling since her early teens. She has had extensive training in dancing and drama, which has been a tremendous asset to her in being selected for special dance scenes in fashion shows. Her ambition is to work behind the scenes in production shows, films, and television. Some of her assignments have been industrial films and commercials for General Electric, Ford, Younger Furriers, TWA, and Renault. She is fully trained to accept any fashion modeling assignment.

ANITA STELLER

House of Charm, San Francisco, California
Age range: 16-21   Hair: Black
Size: 8   Eyes: Hazel
Height: 5 feet 8 inches

Anita is a very natural model. She is completely unaware of herself once she has spent hours preparing for her appearance. Trying new makeup approaches is a hobby. Practicing new ideas from fashion magazines, and inventing a few of her own both in makeup and fashion appeal to her. Top department stores request her often, and she is seen frequently in the local newspapers.

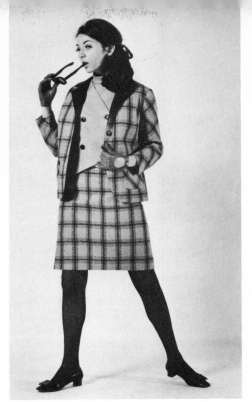

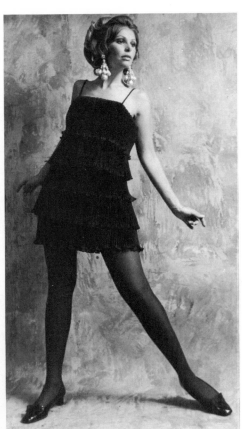

ARLENE TERPSTRA

Vogue Model Agency, Long Beach, California
Age: 20   Hair: Brown
Size: 8-10   Eyes: Blue
Height: 5 feet 11½ inches

A native of California, Arlene is of Dutch descent. She enjoys designing her own clothes, and spends many extra hours sketching. Although she has seriously thought of attending a designing school, at present she is busy with photography assignments. Arlene is especially requested for fur showings. Her ambition is to go to New York and continue her modeling profession.

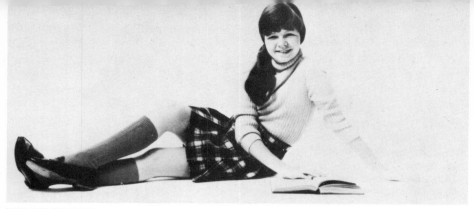

SUSAN TULLY

Dorothy Lohman Model Agency, New York
Age range: 10-14
Size: 10-12 (child); 3-4 (teen)
Height: 5 feet

Hair: Red
Eyes: Blue

Susan Tully started her career at the age of three, modeling for catalogs and magazines such as *Good Housekeeping, Ladies' Home Journal*, and *Parents*. She has thirty-four commercials to her credit, as well as three Broadway plays. Susan takes lessons in ballet, acting, singing, riding, and modeling. She changes with the times, and with each age level that faces her.

She has modeled children's fashions for Lilly Dache, Helen Lee, Kate Greenaway, Youngland, Joseph Love, Cinderella, and scores of other top manufacturers. She follows directions with ease and is every inch a professional.

Her ambition at the moment is to continue working in all phases of modeling and acting. Susan's capabilities assure her of a fine future.

MADY WEIGAND

Frances Gill Model Agency, New York
Age range: 18-25   Hair: Dark blonde
Size: 8-9   Eyes: Blue
Height: 5 feet 7½ inches

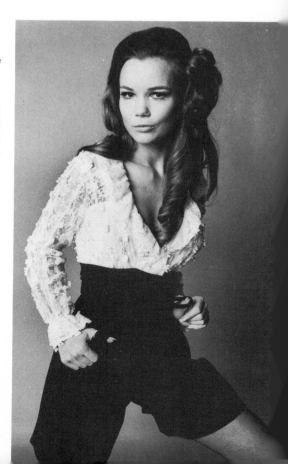

Mady was discovered by Frances Gill while she was modeling at the New York World's Fair in 1964. It was at the fair that she overcame her stage fright. Doing two and three fashion shows daily gave her time to grow in personality and to learn how to project for an audience.

Mady earns approximately $1500 per week doing fashion shows, television, and photography. She is capable of accepting many different assignments.

She is constantly working to improve herself, and often reminisces about the hours spent in practicing her walk and posture. Braces are responsible for her perfect teeth. Model training gave her the foundation for her career. It took almost two years for her to reach the peak of her profession.

Photo by Jordan Flask

14

NECESSARY FORMS AND PROMOTION PIECES

Personal Request Form

When a client hires a model, he must fill out a form, which varies from one agency to another. The model must have a signature stating how many hours she worked and the agreed rate of pay. The client will keep a copy, and the agency will keep a copy. Sometimes the model keeps a third copy for her own record. Model agencies keep a very accurate record of each job for which a model is hired. It is important that all information regarding the assignment be understood and signed for by the client and the agency. Records must be kept carefully for billing and tax purposes.

Wilhelmina MODEL AGENCY INC.	**AGENCY COPY** 527 MADISON AVENUE NEW YORK, N.Y. 10022 Phone: 421-1880	AS AGENT FOR TIME	MODEL	DATE OF JOB
		RATE	R HOUR A T DAY	CLIENT STUDIO / DEPT. OR ACCOUNT
SEND **TO** _____ INVOICE ADDRESS _____ CITY _____ STATE _____			FROM _ _ _ _ _ TO	CHECK FOR FITTING ☐ / TOTAL SUBJECT TO SERVICE CHARGE
NUMBERED COPIES OF THIS INVOICE WILL BE MAILED TO YOU, HOWEVER, IF YOU WISH TO USE THIS INVOICE FOR PAYMENT PLEASE NOTE THE MODEL'S NAME AND DATE OF JOB ON YOUR REMITTANCE.			THE ABOVE WORK HAS BEEN DONE AND THE BILLING INFORMATION IS CORRECT CLIENT'S SIGNATURE _____	
MODEL RELEASE: IN CONSIDERATION OF THE MODEL FEES STATED HEREIN I HEREBY GIVE MY PERMISSION TO THE ABOVE ADVERTISER AND/OR PUBLISHER TO PRODUCE MY PHOTOGRAPH FOR PURPOSES OF ADVERTISING AND/OR TRADE.			MODEL'S SIGNATURE _____	

Request for Models and Personnel

From: Lenz Model Agency
   1456 E. Charleston Blvd.   Telephone
   Las Vegas, Nevada 89104   382-3245

The Lenz Model Agency of Las Vegas, an organization of specially screened and trained personnel in Fashion Models, Exhibit Models, Hostesses, and other specialized personnel. Also Fashion Shows, Tours, and Lectures are arranged for any size group.
The following form is included for your convenience in requesting such personnel. Please fill out carefully and return one copy. Keep one copy for your files.

Please make available _____ personnel. Ages _____

Type _____

Type of apparel _____
         day, evening, special request

Special qualifications or requests _____

_____

_____

Fee per model _____
       Minimum . . . hourly . . . daily

Dates _____

Time schedule A.M. or P.M. _____

Report time _____ Where _____

Person to contact _____

Company or person to be billed

Name _____ Title _____

Address _____

City _____ State _____ Zip _____

Authorized person hiring _____

Lenz Model Agency representative _____

Models hired _____

_____

NEVADA'S ONLY ACCREDITED MODEL AGENCY THROUGH THE MODELING ASSOCIATION OF AMERICA
THIS AGENCY IS LICENSED AND BONDED BY THE LABOR COMMISSIONER OF NEVADA.

Agency Policies

Illustrated is a copy of an agency policy regarding rates and rules. Policies vary in different sections of the country; however, the one printed here prevails in most of the major cities throughout the country.

AGENCY POLICIES: Photography

Day Rates:
A day rate is computed at 5 times the hourly rate and constitutes 8 hours. Anything over 8 hours is regular hourly rate, unless otherwise specified by Agency.

Half-Day:
Half-day rate is computed at 3 times the hourly rate and constitutes 4 hours of the model's time.

All bookings must specify in advance if on an hourly, half-day or day rate. Work booked on an hourly basis cannot be converted to a half-day or day rate after the booking is in progress.

Preparation time:
Prep time is half the hourly rate and can be booked only at the beginning of a booking and must be specified in advance as prep time. This includes only hair, makeup or wardrobe preparation.

Fitting time:
Fitting time is half of the hourly rate, if booked at the beginning of the booking and the minimum is ½ hour.

If booked at a separate time other than at the beginning of the booking the minimum time is one hour.

Travel time:
Travel time is half the hourly rate. Any location where the models use their own car, an additional 10¢ per mile must be included.

Overtime:
Before 6:30 AM and after 6:30 PM is time and one half unless otherwise specified by Agency.

Cancellations:
24 hours prior to booking — no fee.
Less than 24 hours prior to booking — ½ fee.

Weather Permits:
First cancellation for bad weather — no fee.
Second cancellation for bad weather — ½ fee.
Third cancellation for bad weather — full fee.

Editorial Rates:
Unless there is an established rate for magazine, newspaper or trade publication editorial work, the editorial rate is $5.00 less than the regular hourly rate.

Catalogue:
Catalogue rate of $5.00 less per hour may be used only if the booking is for a full day, or more.

Lingerie: Double the hourly rate.

Wardrobe:
If a model is asked to shop for specifics for a booking, preparation time will be charged for the shopping time.

Hand inserts: Full rate.

On experimental and speculation shootings, the models may not sign release unless specific arrangements have been made with the agency, in the event the pictures are sold.

Comps:
Special comp rate may be arranged with the agency.

Background groups:
Special rates may be arranged when a large group of unidentifiable models are to be used in the background.

Products:
Please check with agency for conflict. No bookings for consumers package products may be made without prior clearance with agency.

TV BOOKINGS: On all live and tape bookings which are AFTRA scale or less than 10% over scale, the client must pay the agency commission on original session and any reuse.

Photograph Release

This release is a written agreement between the model and another person stating that the model's picture may be used for any and all purposes in publications and advertising of every description. The other person is usually the photographer, advertiser, or a publisher.

It is wise for a model to remember that she may be signing a complete release which gives the other person the option to use just a portion of her picture in any advertising he may choose. An example would be using a model's body with another model's head, or using a model's picture for a product with which the model would not want to be associated.

There is no need to be concerned about a complete release when you know the people are reputable, and you are protected as an agency model since it is your agency's business to check clients carefully. If in doubt, simply cross out what you do not want in the release and add exactly what picture is to be used and where. The person using your picture must have your signed release to protect him from any lawsuit by you or your agency.

MODEL RELEASE

In consideration of my engagement as a model by

_____ and the receipt by me of $_____,
I hereby give you, those for whom you may be acting, your successors, assigns, licensees and any other designees, forever, the absolute right and permission, throughout the world, to copyright (and to renew and extend any copyright), use, reuse, publish and republish photographic portraits and pictures of me, or in which I may be included, in whole or in part, or composite or distorted in character or form, whether heretofore taken or to be taken in the future, in conjunction with my own or a fictitious or honorary name or title (which I now have or may have in the future) or reproductions thereof, in color or otherwise, made through any media at any place for art, advertising, trade, or any other purpose whatsoever.

I also consent to the use of any printed matter and to giving me, or not giving me, a credit, in the sole discretion of any of the aforementioned parties to whom this authorization and release is given, in conjunction therewith.

I hereby waive any right that I may have to inspect and/or approve the finished product or the advertising copy or printed matter that may be used in connection therewith, or the use to which it may be applied.

I hereby release, discharge and agree to save harmless all the aforementioned parties to whom this authorization and release runs from any liability by virtue of any blurring, distortion, alteration, optical illusion or use in composite form whether intentional or otherwise that may occur or be produced in

the taking of said picture or in any processing tending toward the completion of the finished product, as well as in publication thereof, even though it might otherwise be considered a libel or might subject me to ridicule, scandal, reproach, scorn and indignity.

I hereby represent and warrant that I am of full age and have every right to contract in my own name in the above regard. I state further that I have read the above authorization and release prior to its execution and that I am fully familiar with the contents thereof.

Dated:

_____   _____
Witness

IF MODEL IS A MINOR

We hereby represent that we are the parents and guardians of _____
and that in order to induce you now and in the future to engage him (her) as a model, we hereby irrevocably grant all rights and release from all the liabilities which are the subject of the above "MODEL RELEASE," to all the parties to whom said "MODEL RELEASE" is given. We further state that we have read the aforementioned "MODEL RELEASE" and we are convinced that it is in the best interest of him (her) for said "MODEL RELEASE" to be executed.

Dated:

_____   _____
Witness

Sample Photograph Release

I, _____ , being of legal age hereby

consent and authorize _____

its successors, legal representative and assigns, to use and reproduce my name and

photographs taken by _____ on

_____ and circulate the same for any
and all purposes, including publications and advertising of every description. Consideration is hereby acknowledged, and no further claim of whatsoever nature will be made by
me. No representations have been made to me.

_____

Guardian (if underage)   Model

_____

Witness

_____

Witness

Headsheets

Headsheets are an indispensable part of the modeling picture. They are letter-size sheets of paper with small pictures of models on an entire page. Sometimes an agency will show a head shot (photograph) of a model as well as a body shot of her. More frequently, the agency will have one head shot with the model's statistics under it and occasionally a brief résumé of her past assignments. In any case, headsheets will vary from agency to agency. They are sent out to hundreds of clients who use models, and are kept on file and replaced as new models are added to the files. Headsheets make it easy for a client to select the types of models needed for a specific assignment. Once the client has selected the model or models, he may request more pictures of her, which is where a composite is needed.

Another type of headsheet shows only the head shots of the models, as illustrated. In this type, twenty models can be presented on one page. These headsheets have to be changed every six months to a year to add new faces and use different pictures of the current models for placement.

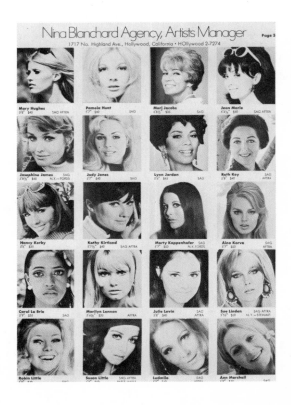

Composites

A composite is a portfolio of photos printed on one sheet. This sheet may be 8½ inches by 11½ inches, or it may be folded into three sections of that size. One-page composites may be paper prints or glossy photographs. Any fold-over type composite is always made in paper-book stock. The composite shows a model in different poses, costumes, moods, and types of assignments for which she would be suitable. It is very important for a model to keep her pictures current and to show at least four different expressions and ways of appearing before a camera. The agency always works closely with its models to help them

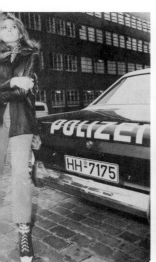
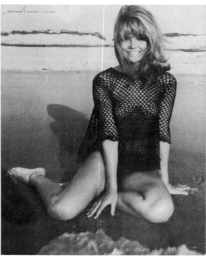
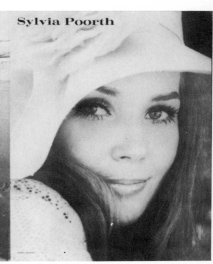
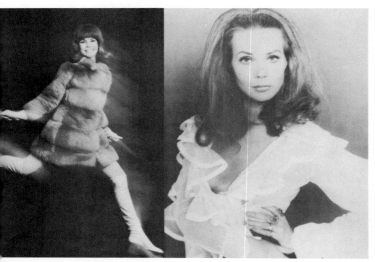
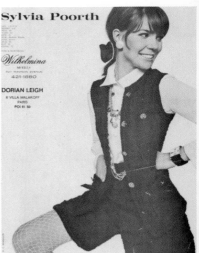

select the best salable pictures for their composites. Although the models pay for the pictures and composites, the best price possible is made available to them by working with their agency.

Another example of composites is shown. Note the different fashions, hairstyles, and moods the model has been careful to use on her composite. This is a four-page composite with one large picture on each page.

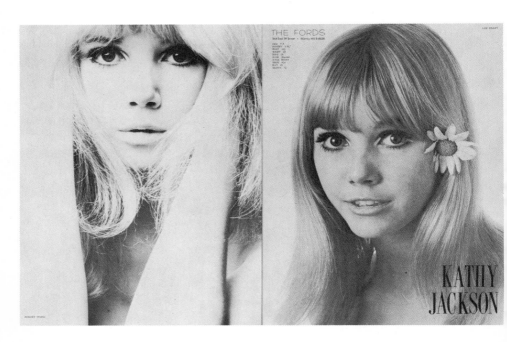

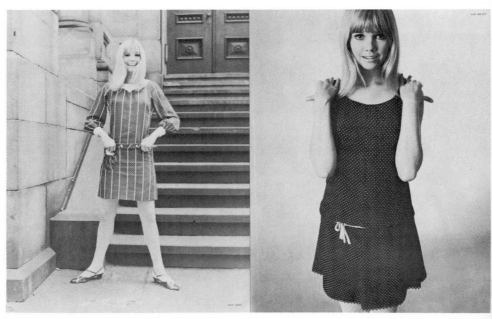

Résumé

When you submit your photograph to a client or an agency, it is good to submit your résumé at the same time. Here is a general outline to follow. You may type the résumés yourself, or if you need many, have a printer make as many copies as you wish.

Sample Résumé

Name—Angelyn Forbes
Age—Ranges from 19 to 25 years (you may give exact age)
Model Agency
    Shore Model Agency, Asbury Park, New Jersey
    Formerly with Frances Gill, New York
Physical Statistics

Height: 5 feet 6 inches	Hair: Dark Brown
Weight: 114 pounds	Eyes: Brown
Bust: 33 inches	Complexion: Medium
Waist: 23 inches	Dress Size: 6, 7, 8
Hips: 34 inches	Shoe: 7½ N

Training—Theatre, Drama, Speech, Wellesley College and University of Rochester
Workshops and Experimental Theatre
    Boston Theatre and Art School
    Harvard School of Drama
    Archibald MacLeish
    Lisa Rauschenbush
    Living Irish Playwrights
Music—Viola and Voice at Eastman School of Music
Dance—Studied under Martha Graham
Member—SAG and AFTRA
Experience
    Theatre—Summer Stock, Rochester, New York—Rochester Music Theatre, general chorus and leads; *Guys and Dolls*—Sarah; *Bye-Bye Birdie*—Rose
    Lecturer, Demonstrator, Convention and Exhibit Model
    Film—Demonstration, Eastman Kodak
      Bausch & Lomb
      Experimental Films
    Television—"New York Illustrated"; "Richard Rodgers Story"
      Fashion Shows
      Commercials: Noreen (hair product), released
        Ultrabrite toothpaste, released
        Lifebuoy Soap
        Hefty Trash Can Liners (voice over)
    Fashion Shows—Stage, Runway, Salon, Wholesale, Tearoom
    Photography—Able to move and project for camera in catalog and editorial assignments.

Doree South

Height—5 feet 10 inches
Weight—125 pounds
Dress—11, 12
Measurements—37—25—37

Eyes—Blue
Hair—Red
Shoe—8½ N
Glove—7½

Modeling

Commercial Photography
  Magazines: *Seventeen, Life, Look, McCall's, Better Homes and Gardens*
  Catalogs: Sears; Advertising Products, etc.

Fashion Shows
  International Designers Show (4 years), Garment Center, and major hotel shows for
  Dresses, Coats, Sportswear, Furs, Bridal, and Lingerie

"17" Model of the Year for T. J. Clothing, representing *Seventeen* magazine. Traveled one
year speaking, commentating, and coordinating shows.

Commercials

General Electric Appliances
Ford (3)
Younger Furriers
TWA
Renault

Industrial Films

National Air Conditioning
General Electric Products
Vogue Films

Industrial Shows

Auto Show; Boat Show; Premium Show; National Farm Machinery Show; National Mobile
Home Show; National Photo Show; Supermarket Show; World's Fair; Spokeswoman
for Kentucky; National Home Furnishings Show; National Postmasters Convention,
Speaker.

Index